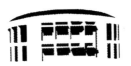
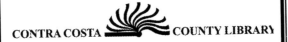

THE NEW SCIENCE
OF PERFECT SKIN

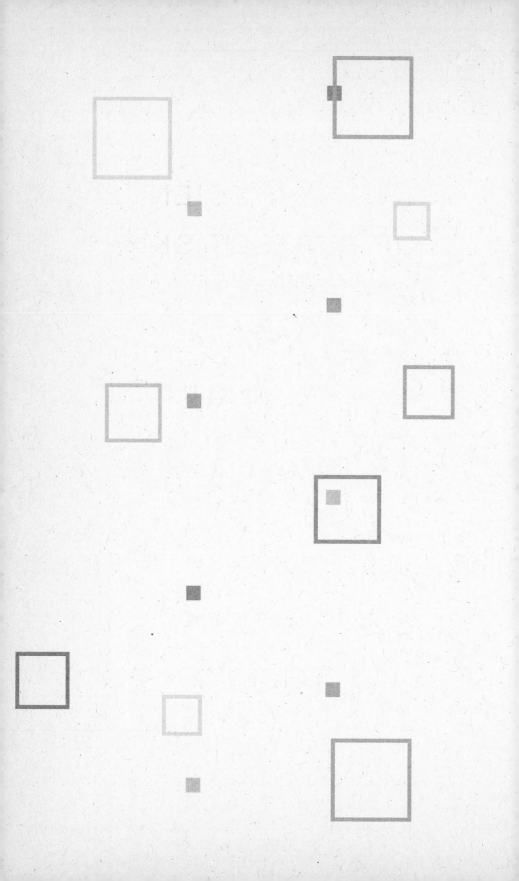

THE NEW SCIENCE
OF PERFECT SKIN

■ ■ ■ ■ ■ ■

Understanding

Skin-Care Myths

and Miracles for

Radiant Skin at Any Age

■ ■ ■ ■

Daniel B. Yarosh, PhD

Broadway Books
New York

BROADWAY

PUBLISHED BY BROADWAY BOOKS

Copyright © 2008 by Dr. Daniel Yarosh

All Rights Reserved

Published in the United States by Broadway Books, an imprint of The
Doubleday Broadway Publishing Group, a division of Random House,
Inc., New York.
www.broadwaybooks.com

BROADWAY BOOKS and its logo, a letter B bisected on the diagonal, are
trademarks of Random House, Inc.

This book is not intended to take the place of medical advice from a
trained medical professional. Readers are advised to consult a physician
or other qualified health professional regarding treatment of their
medical problems. Neither the publisher nor the author takes any
responsibility for any possible consequences from any treatment, action,
or application of a medicine, herb, or preparation to any person reading
or following the information in this book.

Book design by Donna Sinisgalli

Library of Congress Cataloging-in-Publication Data

Yarosh, Daniel.
    The new science of perfect skin : understanding skin-care myths and
miracles for radiant skin at any age / Daniel B. Yarosh. — 1st ed.
        p.   cm.
Includes bibliographical references.
1. Skin—Care and hygiene. 2. Beauty, Personal. 3. Cosmetics.
I. Title.
RL87.Y37 2008
646.7'26—dc22

                                                                2007032677

ISBN 978-0-7679-2539-6

PRINTED IN THE UNITED STATES OF AMERICA

10 9 8 7 6 5 4 3 2 1

First Edition

CONTENTS

■ ■ ■

Acknowledgments   vii

Introduction: Welcome to the New Skin-Care Revolution   1

■ PART I. THE BASICS
1. Skin 101   13

■ PART II. PACKAGING AND INGREDIENTS
2. Cutting Through the Hype   31
3. Your Ingredient Glossary   58

■ PART III. COSMETIC PRODUCTS
4. Cleansers and Toners   83
5. Moisturizers   94
6. Sun Care: It's Never Too Late   117
7. What You Need to Know About Skin Cancer   150
8. Color Changers: Self-Tanners and Lighteners   154
9. Antioxidants and the Emperor's New Clothes   174
10. Wrinkle Treatments   196
11. The Doctor Treatments   217
12. The Future of Skin Care   231

■ PART IV. REGIMENS AND
RECOMMENDATIONS

13. Daily Regimens   243

14. The Master Product List   257

Notes   271

Bibliography   273

Index   285

ACKNOWLEDGMENTS

This book began during a dinner conversation with writer Linda Dyett, and her contributions in editing, suggesting ideas, and overall enthusiastic encouragement have been invaluable in bringing these concepts to life. I owe thanks to publicist Peggy Frank, who arranged that dinner, and literary agents Elisa Petrini, Ryan Fischer-Harbage, Kirsten Neuhaus, and David Vigliano for shepherding me through the publishing process. Karen Moline and Amy Ryan made invaluable contributions in helping me to write and edit so that, I hope, the message gets through. I appreciate Amy Hertz, Sandra Bark, and Ann Campbell at Broadway Books for recognizing that this book might have value for a broad audience.

Physicians and scientists Zoe Draelos, Richard Granstein, Masamitsu Ichihasi, Eric Johansen, Albert Kligman, Hitoshi Masaki, and Ron Moy have offered uninhibited criticism of these ideas to make the book better. Any remaining errors are of course mine alone.

I thank my compatriots in the skin-care business for their encouragement over the years, even when they didn't agree with me: Carol and Steven Kosann, Shigeru Sekine, Herve Offredo, Daniel Maes, Mary Matsui, Tom Mammone, Ken Marenus, Olivier Doucet, Leonhard Zastrow, David Brown, and Marsha Wertzberger.

I am especially grateful to my business colleagues who have supported me whether I was ahead or behind the curve: Jon Klein, Adrienne O'Connor, Matt D'Amico, Nick Bizios, Georgia Binns, Yesenia Plock, Ken Smiles, Fred Carr, Barbara Hayes, Phyllis Dohn, Stan

Nusim, Andrew Fink, Steven Kaye, John Caplan, Tom Pew, Wayne Edwards, Fred Skolnik, Maurice Klee, and all the staff at AGI Dermatics.

Finally, I thank my family, who make this book both possible and worthwhile: my wife, Karen, and children, Haley, Jenna, and Jordan. This book is dedicated to the memory of our founding parents, Norman and Lily Yarosh and William and Sylvia Doninger.

THE NEW SCIENCE
OF PERFECT SKIN

Welcome to the New Skin-Care Revolution

Dermatologists know skin.

But I know *ingredients.*

Over the last thirty years, as an inventor, researcher, manufacturer, supplier, and formulator, I've learned all about the skin-care market from the unique perspective of a practicing scientist. After receiving my doctorate in molecular biology in 1978 from the University of Arizona College of Medicine, I spent seven years at two prestigious research institutes, Brookhaven National Laboratory in New York and the National Cancer Institute in the National Institutes of Health in Bethesda, Maryland, studying how DNA controls the skin's aging process. I then decided to put my knowledge to practical use. With the support of my wife and family, I started up my own biotechnology company, AGI Dermatics, devoted solely to exploring and creating radically different new skin-care ingredients and technology, not only to help prevent skin cancer, but to improve and protect the skin of people of all ages.

These days, the ingredients developed in my lab are found in countless prestige skin-care products around the world, from brands such as Estée Lauder, Coty, and Shiseido. Our own line of Remergent skin-care products is formulated from our cutting-edge ingredients and is sold in dermatologists' offices and in spas and stores across the country and around the world.

Over the last three decades, I've seen changes in the skin-care business that are absolutely astonishing. In fact, I'd say we're in the middle of a New Skin-Care Revolution.

You can understand why I use the word "revolution" if you stop to think about just how dramatically the world of skin care has changed over the last century. Next time you casually apply mascara or dash on a slick of lip gloss, consider that social norms once mandated that makeup was solely worn by stage actresses and ladies of ill repute. Respectable ladies simply did not *do* their faces. And when it came to skin care, "treatments" were limited to moisturizing salves or whitening plasters more likely to harm you than help you. Not surprisingly, cosmetics were typically sold *under* the counter at department stores, and products sold by apothecaries or made at home by countless women remained closely guarded secrets.

The years between the first and second world wars saw an overall change in beauty and fashion thanks to the influences of Hollywood. Studio sets were lit by blazingly hot klieg lights that showcased the slightest of bumps or lines or creases, and directors and cinematographers quickly realized that actors and actresses were in dire need of thick pancake makeup to slather on their faces. Once legitimate actresses began to wear makeup, their fans followed suit, and cosmetics finally began to come out from under the counter. Max Factor, a Russian immigrant, invented formulas especially for the movies, which in turn launched his cosmetic empire. A mixture of five different vegetable oils, developed by a chemist named Alberto for the Culver hairdressing company to protect hair from the harsh lighting, became the very successful Alberto VO5 line of hair care.

During and after World War II, when women began to flock to the workforce, the modern cosmetic industry was launched, with the rise of brands such as Helena Rubinstein, Elizabeth Arden, Estée Lauder, Revlon, and many others. From day one, these brands featured gorgeous advertisements that were cunning enough to promise glamour and youth, but the actual products were designed merely to hide imperfections. We would recognize them today as moisturizers in nice jars. These creams could pump the skin full of water temporarily, but there was no way they could produce sustained benefits. How could they when the technology at the time was limited and there were so few active ingredients available? Even the cosmetic industry elite recognized these products as nothing more than hope in a jar. And for decades, that's just about all women could do—pay for the jars and keep on hoping!

The first wave of the New Skin-Care Revolution began to gather momentum in the 1990s, with the introduction of several new ingredients—alpha-hydroxy acids, retinoic acid (Retin-A), and vitamin A formulations—that really and truly had a measurable impact on skin. These were followed by advancements in chemical peels and lasers, then a whole new category of injectable substances like Botox and fillers, all of which delivered immediate benefits that lasted longer than a scant few hours. These new ingredients and procedures actually made changes in the skin by clearing away its debris, temporarily relaxing muscles, or by filling in troughs and wrinkles. Because they worked so quickly and so dramatically (making them beloved by many in Hollywood), they set a standard for fast and visible results that all products have been held to ever since. For the first time in history, women could witness their complexions becoming smoother, firmer, more buoyant, less wrinkled, less mottled—rejuvenated, in fact. It was as if the clock could be turned back twenty years.

Perhaps those who like to joke that fifty is the new forty, or that sixty is the new fifty, aren't kidding after all. A whopping 78 million Americans will begin turning 65 in 2011. This baby boomer generation is living longer and better than previous generations, growing older in good physical and mental health and feeling and acting much younger than the calendar says—and they demand that their skin-care products *work*. Luckily, we live in an era when their demands can be met—if they learn what products to buy for their skin, as well as how to use them.

Today, we are entering what I call the New Skin-Care Revolution, with third-millennium treatments and ingredients, many of which are either just becoming available or are set to launch within the next few years. These products don't just remove surface damage but actually reprogram the skin's natural functioning at the cellular level. Even if you shudder when you think back to your high school science classes, it's not hard to understand why reprogramming the skin's natural functioning is a truly revolutionary concept. These third-millennium products focus on the interaction of genes and are guided by recent breakthroughs in our understanding of the human DNA code, or genomics. That's what I mean by the "new science of perfect skin."

Throughout this book, I'll give you an overview of the new tools derived from genetic science—tools that, for the first time, can truly repair and even reverse the signs of aging. You'll learn more about the growing arsenal of new ingredients such as endonucleases, retinol, and phytoestrogens, which have been shown to fine-tune the skin's inner workings—its very metabolism, in fact—in order to protect, energize, and reinvigorate skin, not for a few hours or a few days or even a few months, but for years to come. These remarkable new ingredients—the first ever to be based on our new knowledge of DNA, human genomics, and photobiology (the science of the effects of sunlight, especially ultraviolet light, on life)—can radically change the way your skin looks and functions. And they will radically change the way skin-care products are conceived.

And so, this book is indeed about a New Skin-Care Revolution— the newest wave in an ongoing story of beauty, elevated to the next level by molecular science. Our fundamental understanding of how the skin ages has undergone a quantum shift, and the new biology is making way for a new kind of skin care. These fantastic new ingredients and the technology that can deliver them, backed by rigorous scientific testing and compelling evidence of their success, have just one goal in mind: perfect skin. Skin that is clear, smooth, and supple. Skin that looks and acts young again. Skin that *stays* young.

Today, there are products that really work. That's the good news. Now here's the bad news—and the reason why you need this book! Despite the gains made by the New Skin-Care Revolution, there's never been more confusion and uncertainty about which products get results and which are a waste of money and time.

The skin-care business is an economic powerhouse—a $15 billion anti-aging and rejuvenation industry. But it is also an industry bloated by an incredible array of companies and products, each touting itself as the newest, best, most radical, and most worthy of your loyalty. Of course, some of these companies spend tens of millions of dollars each year in research and product development, stay abreast of the newest trends, seek out important discoveries, and use only the most efficacious ingredients in their products. Some of these are tiny companies driven by the desire to improve skin and keep it looking good, who sell their products by word of mouth, while others are global brands with enormous advertising budgets.

And so consumers are bombarded by enticing ads featuring models and celebrities with creamy, flawless skin; ever-so-helpful salesclerks spouting pseudoscience at the cosmetics counters; and countless articles in women's magazines puffing up the Very Best New Thing on a monthly basis. So how do you know what really works?

Few consumers really understand what, precisely, is inside each jar of cream that they buy and why it's supposed to improve their skin. Or what kind of packaging enhances the product inside and what doesn't. Or why some serums and lotions are astonishingly expensive yet in truth not worth a fraction of their cost. Which products really deliver on their promises? The high-tech ones? Those costing the equivalent of a week's salary? The dermatologists' brands? The major prestige and mass-market brands, backed by the kind of research only large corporations can afford? The botanical lines? The esoteric French or Japanese imports? The back-to-basic folk remedies?

What about the major brands that tell women they need to use an entire line of single-purpose cosmetics for weeks on end in order to see results? Or the saleswomen who insist that you simply *must* buy one cream to minimize pores, another to tone under your chin, yet another to remove dark circles under your eyes, and a fourth to lift sagging eyelids? Or the brands that feature endless variations on a theme, each with the same ingredients but in the form of a lotion, serum, gel, cream, or tonic, one for morning, one for evening, and one for use only around the eyes? And don't forget the creams to repair, clarify, hydrate, relax, and stimulate!

Choosing skin-care products has become incredibly confusing. And what makes this confusion so annoying is the fact that while there are terrific new high-tech products that didn't exist a few years ago, they're stocked on the shelves alongside the well-known old-school products that are next to the cosmeceuticals and organic and holistic products. All of them are smartly packaged and loaded with enticing claims, but only some of them work.

I don't mean to imply that the cosmetics industry as a whole is out to dupe consumers. Some companies might be, but most aren't. There are a lot of incredibly good products out there, especially products of the New Skin-Care Revolution, that dramatically improve your skin and make it feel amazingly fine. Some even give better results than expected. But they are trying to make their voices heard in an enormous and very noisy marketplace well known for pushing myths, glitz, and hype.

Consumers shopping for treatment products have more choices than ever before, and they don't care where they buy these products—whether from dermatologists, cosmetic counters, the Internet, drugstores, specialty stores, infomercials, or the door-to-door salesperson—but they do care if these products work. I'd say that many consumers are frustrated and skeptical, if not downright cynical, about many of the claims they see on the packages. Without question, consumers have been let down by some ad claims, and by beauty magazines and television shows that have failed to serve as consumer advocates and haven't asked the critical questions needed to sort through so much hard sell and hype.

Compounding the problem presented by so many choices is the convergence of dermatology and cosmetics. Dermatologists and plastic surgeons are performing cosmetic procedures, such as the use of injectable fillers, Botox, laser treatments, chemical peels, and microdermabrasion and other exfoliating techniques, in their offices at unprecedented rates. They're also recommending specific products and even developing and marketing their own skin-care collections. At the same time, cosmetic companies are touting the virtues of their easily available over-the-counter products and positioning them as far less expensive alternatives to invasive or painful medical procedures. For the first time ever, doctors and cosmetic companies are literally competing with each other to treat the same concerns about aging skin! And their clientele has changed from patients to consumers of health-care products—consumers who still have more questions than answers.

So how can you cut through this dazzling display of cosmetic confusion?

I'm going to tell you how.

The goal of *The New Science of Perfect Skin* is to answer the question every skin-care consumer asks: What works and what doesn't?

Because I understand skin-care products from the inside out, I can separate fact from myth, help from hype, and gems from junk and let you know what has been overpraised and what has been overlooked. In part 1, I'll give you a short primer on skin so you can understand how DNA controls the way it ages and what can be done about it. In part 2, I'll show you how to cut through the cosmetic-industry hype, giving you the tools you'll need to sort through the claims and help you make smart choices whenever you shop for effective skin-care cosmetics. You'll be able to judge product claims effectively and decipher ingredient labels. I'll also set the record straight with specifics about the broad range of brand-new, not-so-new, and classic cosmetics and cosmeceutical ingredients, both lab created and botanically based, and how well they really work.

In part 3, I'll take an in-depth look at the New Skin-Care Revolution products that you need—and the products you don't. I'll be naming names and telling the tales of products that deliver and those that are little more than a puff of smoke and a funhouse mirror. Once I explain what DNA reprogramming and repair are—the true breakthroughs in today's skin-care science and techniques that can truly rejuvenate skin—you'll be able to know what new products are available and will be able to see through the propaganda and exaggerated promises of a marketplace that has needed this examination for far too long. You'll learn that the best new and effective skin treatments have nothing to do with fad diets, rare natural botanicals from exotic locales, or "Eureka!" moments from maverick dermatologists with improbable new discoveries of this or that "miraculous" ingredient—all of which have somehow passed over the hard-core scientific proof of how these products work!

If you're in your twenties and thirties, you'll learn how wrinkles, sagging, and age spots can be simply and easily prevented from forming in the first place, and as a result, you can kick the Botox-and-Restylane habit before it even starts. Those age forty and beyond will learn to use DNA repairing and reprogramming products so that it's not too late to

---

Luxury and Drugstore Products

Throughout the book I denote luxury products with a ❋ and drugstore products with a •.

Luxury products (❋) are those that are high-priced (usually more than $40 a bottle) and are found at department store cosmetic counters, specialty stores, or on the Internet. They usually have limited distribution.

Drugstore products (•) are those that are more moderately priced (usually under $40 a bottle) and are widely found in chain drugstores, supermarkets, mass-market stores like Wal-Mart and Target, television shopping shows, and from personal sales companies like Amway, Avon, and Mary Kay.

The ways cosmetic products are sold are changing rapidly, and there are no hard and fast rules about where products may be found. These are only guidelines to help you locate the products you want.

---

undo the skin damage sustained in youth. And women of all ages will learn how to reduce skin inflammation—from the sun, from the elements, from stress and overindulgent lifestyles—which is the key to perfectly healthy skin. I'll also take a peek into what products of the future might look like.

In part 4, you'll find everything you need to take care of your skin, including a master list of some of the best skin-care products currently available. I'll also show you exactly how to use them with a few simple and effective beauty regimens, so that your skin will look its very best, no matter what your calendar age.

The products created by the New Skin-Care Revolution will make taking care of your skin easier instead of more complex. You'll be able to streamline your daily skin-care routine and cut out the vast array of single-purpose cosmetics, because you'll be using "smart" products with multiple active ingredients. Happily for you, the time is coming when women of any age will need only three or four basic products to achieve the best skin of their lives.

Once you've been armed with my smoking guns, I hope that you'll never again fall for any hype and that you'll be able to demand, with complete confidence, not only "How much, how fast?" but also "Where's the proof?" My ultimate goal is to help you slow down the aging process altogether, so that your skin can remain unchanged once you

Product Recommendations

Throughout the book and particularly in chapter 14, "The Master Product List," I make product recommendations that I base on the ingredients listed on the packaging and inserts, on my own experience and testing, and on the best available information from the manufacturer, the beauty magazines and books, and the scientific literature. It is not possible, of course, to test every product in a double-blind, placebo-controlled study (you'll find out more about that type of study in chapter 2). Often the type of information I would like to have, such as the percent of the ingredient in the product or the chemical composition of the extract, is simply not available, so in those cases I consider what is known about the ingredients by molecular biologists and cosmetic chemists, the reputation of the manufacturer and marketer, and reviews of the product in print and on the Web. Since there are no precise testing rules, I list the recommended products in alphabetical order (not in any ranking of potency). In some cases, the manufacturer changed the name slightly from the time I tested it. In other cases whole product lines have sprung from a single product I examined. I recommend more than one product in each category for many reasons: no one product suits everyone's preference for scent, color, or feel; often several products perform about the same; and sometimes less expensive products are nearly as good as or even better than the expensive ones. In a very few cases, such as some antioxidant products and cleansers with additives, I recommend products that have some suspect or overrated ingredients (I try to make that clear when I do) because they have other very beneficial ingredients and they have some redeeming features (such as a nice texture)—they won't hurt you, but you might be paying for some things you don't need. My purpose is to help you narrow down the choices to just a few products that work, not to give you an iron-clad instruction manual. Remember, there is no substitute for trying the products to find the ones you like and that work for you!

reach your early thirties—and for decades to follow. Instead of seeming to age overnight, you'll find yourself with fresh and natural beauty that unfolds ever so slowly. Instead of being a woman of a certain age, you'll be a woman of an indeterminate age who has never looked better. Welcome to the New Skin-Care Revolution!

PART I

■ ■ ■ ■ ■ ■

THE BASICS

■   ■   ■

ONE

Skin 101

Along with the rest of the body, human skin has evolved over roughly 7,500 generations, give or take a few. These genetically driven changes have been fueled over the millennia by selection for what is optimal for one thing and one thing only: sex.

Yes, that's right: sex, as in human reproduction.

Biologically speaking, skin has the same ultimate purpose as the rest of the human body: contributing to the continuation of the species. As a result, the genes that were passed down to you and everyone you know are the good ones that produced healthy and glowing skin, protected the body, and, most of all, attracted a mate. The bad skin genes that caused disease, weakened the individual, and turned off potential partners didn't get passed on and were eventually lost from the gene pool.

The way people look during the different stages of life fits in with this biological imperative. A baby's skin is soft and smooth to encourage its mother to care for it. During puberty, skin may look aggravated, angry, and out of sorts—which it is. But it's just adapting like the rest of the body to the surge of hormones and physical changes that transform children into adults. (This is, not surprisingly, little consolation to a teenager who suddenly develops terrible breakouts!)

From a biological point of view, the childbearing years are when skin really counts, as people who look their best are much more likely to attract a mate. Those with clear, radiant skin get the highest marks in the gene-pool competition, so it's no wonder that the skin's genetic program is designed to reach a crescendo of health and fitness during the courtship and reproduction years. In most cases, skin in the twenties and early thirties doesn't require much more than cleansing, moisturizing, and daily protection from the sun. Remember, these are the years that generations of human evolution have selected for maximum health with minimum maintenance.

Skin genes controlling shape and texture are not the only determining factor of who beds down with whom, of course, but during the mating ritual, they provide, often unconsciously and in a single glance, an enormous amount of information. A man looking at a woman will make instant judgments about her overall health, fitness, and the degree to which she possesses the "it" factor known as sex appeal. At the same time, a woman is also gathering vital information from her instant judgment about a man's looks. This was proven by a recent study at the University of California, Santa Barbara, which found that women can identify those men with higher testosterone levels and select those with high paternal quality and those who especially like infants just by looking at photographs of the men's faces.

Bottom line: Skin was built for sex. Skin health peaks during the reproductive years; after that, we need help.

THE SKIN YOU'RE IN

Your skin is a whole lot more than an inert overcoat, or something you might think of as cellular Saran wrap. It's a living thing—the largest organ of your body and one that changes dynamically over the course of your lifetime.

Like most organs, skin has two main layers: the dermis, the thick layer on the bottom; and the epidermis, the thin layer of cells on the surface above.

The living dermis is mainly comprised of cells called fibroblasts. These fibroblasts are surrounded by collagen and elastin fibers to form the stretchy supporting structure of the skin. The dermis is also infused with blood vessels to supply nutrients and take away waste, as well as nerves for exquisitely delicate sensation. Hair and oil and sweat glands are all anchored in the dermis and poke or wind their way out to the surface.

Perched on top of the dermis is the epidermis, a layer no more than about twenty cells deep. The cells making up this layer are called keratinocytes. They divide rapidly, but they only grow up, never down. As a result, whenever a keratinocyte divides, the newer cell is always on top. Think of this process as if the bottom cells are the grandmothers, and they divide into daughter cells that in turn divide into a new generation of daughter cells. All this continual division pushes the daughters, the granddaughters, and great-granddaughters up to the surface. It takes about two weeks for newly created daughter cells to be pushed to the surface, where they're sloughed off.

The very outermost layers of skin are stacked atop one another like shingles on a roof. After all the daughter cells finish dividing and reach the top of the skin surface, they flatten out, creating an intercellular cement mixture where ceramides and other lipids connect them to one another. Ceramides are lipids, a type of oil chemical. Each ceramide molecule has two ends, and each end can bind to other chemicals so that a long chain, or mesh, is formed. This network of mesh is what binds the flattened cells together to become the part of the outer skin barrier known as the stratum corneum.

The stratum corneum is basically dead skin cells, but it still serves an extremely vital function: preventing water from escaping from the skin. Without the barrier of the stratum corneum, essential water would evaporate from your body like steam from a boiling kettle, and you would dry up like a raisin in a few hours. The stratum corneum barrier also keeps out invaders, like deadly bacteria and viruses. The barrier function of the stratum corneum is literally a matter of life and death.

During the entire process of forming the dermis, epidermis, and stratum corneum, skin cells undergo a remarkable, genetically programmed transformation. Our genetic code, which exists in our DNA, tells our cells what to do. This is the DNA program.

The DNA program is like a computer program—a series of instructions about what to do and when to do it, intended to be performed in an orderly fashion. A person's DNA program tells a cell when to make things or how to act, as well as how to change what it is doing as it gets older or how to react when it gets information from other cells.

As in a computer program, if a DNA instruction is changed, the cell behaves differently. If the cell gets signals from damaged skin, or by the inevitable aging process itself, it can follow a new course of steps that are harmful to the skin. However, if we introduce special ingredients that give out new signals, we can reprogram the cell to change its course of development and change its function. This transformation, which is directed by information coded in the human genome, is the key to the New Skin-Care Revolution.

Bottom line: The skin has several parts and is constantly changing under the direction of its DNA program.

HOW SKIN CHANGES AS YOU AGE

Until now, aging was pretty much a steady downhill slide. Each month past those prime childbearing years seemed to add a new wrinkle and furrow, a little more drooping and sagging, strange new blotches and uneven tone, and more than a smattering of dark spots that can no longer be thought of as cute little freckles. Before you blame your parents or too frequent beach vacations, realize that both are culprits, because there are two basic ways the skin ages: intrinsic and extrinsic.

Intrinsic aging is driven by the genetic code, and up until now this has been pretty much out of your control. Intrinsic aging follows a specific process:

- The outer barrier weakens
- DNA repair lessens
- Blood flow declines
- Collagen degrades
- Chronic inflammation flares

Further, the underlying fat that gives us such delicious chubby cheeks as children is absorbed, so faces look more gaunt, the bones thin, and the muscles supporting the skin weaken. Then gravity takes over and jowls form, lips thin, cheekbones jut out, earlobes sag, noses seem to grow longer, and tiny blood vessels suddenly appear on the skin's surface.

Extrinsic aging is caused by factors you can control. This includes the devastating effects of the sun upon skin, called photoaging. Photoaging is without question the largest extrinsic factor affecting your skin, causing it to get thick, rough, wrinkled, mottled, flaky, saggy, and covered with spots and uneven pigmentation. I can tell people till I'm blue in the face that there's no such thing as a healthy tan—but getting them to act like it is another issue altogether! Photoaging is the easiest extrinsic factor you can control, and it's never too late to start protecting your skin from the sun.

How to protect yourself from photoaging and the effects of the sun is so crucial that I've devoted an entire chapter to it. Chapter 6 is a primer on photoaging, sunscreen and sun protection, and DNA repair and is without doubt the most important chapter in the book.

Other extrinsic factors are smoking, poor nutrition, stress, not getting enough sleep, and in general taking your skin for granted. The temptation is to play today and pay tomorrow, but it's never too early to start protecting your skin—*now.*

Bottom line: Aging is caused by both your genes and your behavior.

AGING IN THE CHILDBEARING YEARS

Of all the stages of life, the childbearing years put the greatest strain on the body and the skin. Once a woman has reached the peak of her health and attractiveness, she is now subjected to the toughest challenge of all—preparing for and giving birth to children. During this time, sensitivity to sun and irritants increases just as the damage accumulated from the childhood years begins to appear. On top of that, in the thirties, the production of skin lipids begins to decline, weakening the skin barrier.

The childbearing years usually find women in their healthy prime, but it is during this time, when a woman seems to need it least, that the biggest gains can be made in fighting aging. A little understanding of the changes driven by genes and hormones can help any woman preserve her most youthful looks.

For women in their twenties and thirties, many problems related to dryness, irritation, and acne are caused by hormonal changes during their monthly cycle. In the weeks prior to menstruation, the skin's barrier is the weakest and sun sensitivity is the greatest, so extra care should be taken to moisturize, wear sunscreen, and reduce sun exposure. During and after her period, a woman's skin is the most dry and the most sensitive, which calls for careful cleansing (see chapter 4) as well as continued moisturizing with a product containing an anti-irritating, calming agent (see chapter 5).

Pregnancy causes a massive surge in the hormones estrogen and progesterone and can cause visible and often embarrassing changes in the skin. These usually come in the form of dark spots, acne, and/or discolored patches, a form of hyperpigmentation called chloasma, or "the mask of pregnancy," which usually fades after childbirth (a range of brightening and lightening options, covered in chapter 8, can help). Stretch marks may appear, a result of the distension and contraction of pregnancy that leave the abdominal muscles weak and skin paper thin. Add to that the irregular sleep, exhaustion, and the stresses of parenting, and a mother's good looks are never so challenged.

Bottom line: The childbearing years are when you look your best and also when your skin faces its greatest challenges.

CHANGE IN MIDDLE AGE

After the age of thirty-five and into the forties is an ideal time for a woman to find a serious skin protection and reprogramming regimen that will slow aging to a crawl. This is where the products from the New Skin-Care Revolution can have their greatest benefit.

Even though we are living longer and with healthier bodies than ever before, and even though enormous social changes have led to many people no longer being defined by age but by their stage in life, DNA just doesn't care. You might be forty-six and look thirty, but you can't fool your DNA. So even if at forty-six you've just run your twentieth marathon, your peak reproductive years are long gone, and the genetic program dictating changes in your skin has begun to run out of code.

Around the age of forty, our DNA instructions for renewing and rejuvenating our skin essentially stop. The pressure for survival is at its peak during the childbearing years, so as far as our DNA is concerned, once we've successfully produced the next generation, our job is done. Evolution just hasn't kept up with the social changes and improvement in medical care and nutrition that allow so many of us to live decades longer than human beings once did. As a result, your cells' ability to repair DNA damage begins to diminish sometime in the twenties, and by the time you reach age seventy about half of this defense system is lost.

In addition, during the thirties, the skin gradually loses its barrier function. This begins when the production of ceramides is reduced. Ceramides, remember, are those essential oils that hold the stratum corneum layer together like glue. Fewer ceramides means a reduction in the stratum corneum's strength. (By the age of sixty, ceramides have been so depleted that a third of the skin's barrier defense has been lost.)

During your forties, your skin changes dramatically. The decline in DNA repair paves the way for collagen breakdown and the first deep wrinkles. Those days of unprotected sunning now show up as flaky patches and spots that are either overpigmented or underpigmented. Couple that with reduced estrogen levels as menopause approaches, which in turn diminishes collagen, diminishing skin's strength, and there's not only a weakening of the outer innate defenses against toxins from the environment, but also a compromising of the foundation of underlying collagen and elastin. The result? Fine lines, wrinkles, sags, creases, and less elasticity.

While all this is going on, your skin is also losing about 35 percent of its antioxidant vitamin reservoir. The enzymes that initiate inflammatory responses begin to increase, and the blood flow to the skin declines. This means that the skin becomes more sensitive, cooler to the touch, blotchy, and more easily irritated and inflamed.

Like it or not, by the time you hit forty, skin health is as big an issue as skin beauty. Ignore it at your peril!

Bottom Line: Aging begins to appear in the forties when the genetic program has run out of instructions, and skin is left without a regeneration program.

THE YOUNG OLD

More and more people are living well beyond the official age that senior discounts and Social Security kick in. In fact, those in the sixty-five to seventy-four age group now constitute such a clear-cut new contingent that they are being called the "young old."

Women who are over the age of sixty today are the lost beauty generation—the last generation to come of age before the era of the New Skin-Care Revolution. Of course, many mature women who practiced safe sun, used Retin-A early on, or inherited hardworking anti-aging genes have retained their clear, buoyant complexions. But for the most part, these women have skin that's been left to its own devices. If you're over sixty and you feel that you've missed the boat, there's good news— you haven't!

At sixty-five, women experience more than just skin changes; the skin is actually restructuring. Along with problems of bone resorption, there is a loss of the fat that fills out the "apples" of our cheeks, as well as the neck, temples, and the area around the lips. The changes noticed in middle age, such as slight wobbles, become larger sags, and smile lines and lines between the nose and top lip become permanent. Skin is blotchy, dull, and gray. It loses its vitality. It's dry and flaky. It looks, well, *old*.

Many women, refusing to live with the sags and wrinkles and dry skin, have taken a decidedly proactive stance to combat aging. They know the results that injectables such as Botox and fillers can deliver, diminishing wrinkles and replacing lost volume and filling in lines. They know that lasers, peels, and cosmetic surgery can reinvigorate the outer layers of skin, recontour the face, and restore a healthy, youthful, and attractive appearance.

All of these approaches, however, treat older skin as a stone to be sculpted and painted. The New Skin-Care Revolution uses a completely different tactic. Even those who've reached the young-old years can benefit by protecting their delicate skin from the sun, repairing damage, and moisturizing. They still need to augment their DNA repair, increase their microcirculation to warm the skin and heal from cosmetic procedures, and make more ceramides to glue together the outer layer of skin.

In other words, it's time to give their skin new instructions and direction toward rejuvenation. And if they supplement this DNA reprogramming with specific skin-care products designed to address specific problems like age spots, dark under-eye circles, and irritable skin, it's pretty amazing how young the young old can really look.

Bottom line: Seniors face big changes in their skin, but the new advances in the skin-care revolution really work to restore youthful looks.

DON'T FORGET THE OLDEST

I have seen eighty-year-old women with an undeniable beauty that overshines the imperfections of age. But instead of being venerated, those who've reached old age in our society are often discounted and dismissed, especially where their appearance is concerned. Even the New Skin-Care Revolution has, to its shame, largely ignored the skin-care requirements of those in their seventies and older. This needs to be rectified, as those over seventy-four belong to the fastest-growing population group today, with many now living into their nineties and longer.

At this age, skin is extremely thin, dry, and fragile, with little elasticity. It needs special attention and extra hydration, especially for those who suffer from circulatory disorders, diabetes, and hypertension, all of which make bleeding more likely and slow down skin healing. It's more crucial than ever to keep skin completely protected from sun exposure, as precancerous conditions as well as skin cancers are very common. Luckily, there should be skin-care products especially for geriatric skincare arriving in the next decade. They are long overdue.

Bottom line: New products for elderly skin are on the way.

STRESS AND THE SKIN

The way we feel is reflected in the way we look: stress shows in your skin. All you have to do is take a look at the grey-tinged pallor of college students cramming for exams to see what stress has done to their faces. Their skin pretty closely resembles the ash on the cigarettes they know they shouldn't be smoking.

Molecular biologists have recently learned how profoundly stress affects the way you look. The skin's topmost layers are chock-full of astonishingly sensitve nerve endings, and they have a dramatic effect on the skin's appearance. These nerve endings send out tiny chemicals, called neurotransmitters, which tell neighboring cells—whether nerve, skin, blood, or immune cells—that a nerve signal has been received. Excessive release of neurotransmitters suppresses the immune system and constricts blood flow, resulting in the sallow, tired skin we recognize in anxious friends and overtaxed coworkers. (Try telling that to the companies producing dermatologist formulas, such as N.V. Perricone, MD, that want to *add* neurotransmitters to your skin!)

In clinical studies, stress has also been associated with poor functioning of the skin barrier against outside insults. A person under stress, such as at a job interview, has a huge spike in water loss from the skin as the barrier function collapses. Couples who fight have measurably reduced skin immune system function compared to happily married couples! You can't fool the skin. It's a highly sensitive portal that reveals exactly what's going on inside.

To make matters worse, stress can also crank up other skin responses. Most patients with psoriasis, for example, report that stress aggravates their disease. Recent research has even shown that stress raises the level of skin cancer in animals. We are only just beginning to understand the influence of nerves and stress on skin, but until it is better understood, it makes sense to minimize stress because it wreaks havoc on your skin as well as your emotions.

Bottom line: Lifestyle stress has proven negative effects on skin.

DIET AND THE SKIN

Common sense suggests that your diet has an impact on your appearance and the quality of your skin, but science isn't quite sure exactly how. And it isn't always as easy to see the effects as you might think.

Certainly, in extreme cases of vitamin or nutrient insufficiency, a correct diagnosis can be made at a single glance by skilled eyes. But the impact of subtler differences in nutrition has been very difficult to measure quantitatively and definitively. Several recent and highly publicized studies have failed to show the clear link between changing diet and improving health.

So what exactly are we supposed to eat to help our skin look its best? There is no doubt that eating a healthy, balanced diet full of vegetables and fruit and low in saturated fat protects a body against heart disease and cancer. But antioxidant supplements have not had the same success, which only serves to show us that we don't know exactly what's in these delicious vegetables and fruits that makes them so beneficial. (We'll look more closely at this surprising conclusion in chapter 9.) And although we've all been told about "good" cholesterol and "bad" cholesterol and the kind of fats that can lead to higher cholesterol levels, a comprehensive study in 2006 by the Women's Health Initiative of more than 48,000 women on normal or low-fat diets failed to show dramatic changes in the rate of cardiovascular disease, strokes, breast cancer, or colorectal cancer in those who stuck to a low-fat diet. This same study also failed to find benefits for vitamin E, an antioxidant vitamin long thought to have restorative health effects.

Some proponents of low-fat or high-in-antioxidant diets try to blame the patient and not the cure, claiming that the participants either didn't follow the diet or didn't cut down enough on fat. But those expectations are totally unrealistic. It's true that America has become a nation of the overweight, and it's a distressing fact that we're only getting fatter every day. But any diet that expects women to starve themselves is a diet doomed to failure. Solutions that people can't or won't maintain are no solutions at all.

A better understanding of basic human genetics might help explain what kind of diet is best for human bodies. Due to a lot of overly simplified storytelling, many people have come to believe that there was one way of eating that was "natural" for all humans. As a result, many believe that there is one "natural" healthy diet that should be eaten if we want to become and stay healthy and vigorous. This belief may, in fact, not be true at all. When modern humans migrated out of Africa, they quickly expanded to all corners of the earth, including some places where there was no whole grain bread, lean beef, or gardens full of sprouts and leafy greens! Luckily, humans are omnivorous—we can eat just about anything, and each group of people around the globe has its distinct diet, with its own mix of fat, protein, carbohydrates, fiber, and sugars. People with beautiful skin have been raised on each of these many different diets.

Bottom line: There is no such thing as one "natural" diet for all people, and perfect skin does not depend on any one diet in particular.

THE FAT GENES

What we can say with complete confidence is that the one characteristic that's the same for all humans, no matter what their race, where they live, or what they eat, is that we're not built for the good times but to survive the bad ones. Our ancestors were the humans who survived and reproduced when times were tough, when the rain didn't fall, the fish weren't biting, and the herds were thin.

In our modern society where food is abundant, the genetic predisposition to store fat is not such a great thing; the body doesn't know that the supermarket will be open tomorrow. The continual eating of excessive carbohydrates puts extra demands on insulin to store this food as fat. This may very well be one of the primary reasons for the rapidly increasing incidence of diabetes in America and other countries with an abundance of food.

For now, that is what we know for sure. Scientists who are trying to understand the mechanisms of longevity are studying molecular biology—looking precisely at how our genes influence aging. Until all these mechanisms are better understood, the best way to keep your skin looking good is to

■ Eat a diet balanced with a variety of proteins and carbohydrates. Vegetarians must be especially vigilant because many vegetables don't contain all of the nutrients essential for good health, such as omega-3 oils from fish.

■ Reduce your sugar intake, including alcohol, bread, and sweet fruits.

■ Forget drinking gallons of water every day. There is no real clinical evidence that consuming the standard regimen of at least eight glasses of water each day does anything special for skin.

■ Remember that the best diet will always be one filled with whole foods you carefully control by cooking yourself, so that you ingest the most potent vitamins and minerals and nutrients, and that you can cook with the least amount of fats and added sugar.

■ Understand that you don't need to supplement your diet with bottles full of nutritional supplements, because megadoses don't seem to work. Get the right amount of vitamins from a single daily vitamin supplement and leave the rest alone!

Bottom line: Don't be taken in by the hype of unproven, fad beauty diets; there is very little evidence that they affect the skin in any way.

THE GENETICS OF SKIN AGING— REPROGRAMMING THE SKIN

When you look in the mirror, do you see your mother staring back at you? Is your hair the same curly red as your father's? Do you have the same milky white skin as your great-aunt or the luscious honey hues of your grandmother?

All of us resemble our ancestors in some way, and it doesn't take a Nobel Prize in genetics to understand why. Our appearance is controlled by our genes, and we get our genes from our parents. As new babies are born to each subsequent generation, the set of genes coded by our familial DNA dictates that the same color of skin and eyes and hair will appear over and over again, in a precise program that unfolds from birth and continues over a person's life. At each generation, the DNA from both the mother and the father reach a kind of agreement, and then they pass the information on via an unfolding construction program. Ninety-nine percent of our DNA is shared by all humans, and we all have common DNA codes for the same body plan. These direct the way in which we are born, develop, and mature—and the way our skin ages.

Advances in molecular biology, including the Human Genome Project, which cracked the code that makes us human, have turned the way we understand how skin changes from birth to senior citizenship completely upside down. The old-school theory stated that the skin was like a magic, shape-shifting overcoat. It grew as we did, accumulating damage along the way—cuts and scrapes in childhood, one too many sunburns—and general wear and tear in the adult years until finally it just wore out. But the New Skin-Care Revolution sees skin not only as a dynamic organ regenerating itself every day, but also as one that re-makes itself over a lifetime. Since the DNA in our genes is programmed to make specific changes in our skin at specific times, by using the right products, applied at the right time, you can stall, stop, and even *reverse* some of these transformations.

As we've learned, your skin's appearance is the result of both what the environment has done to it (extrinsic factors), and what your DNA has told it to do (intrinsic factors). These extrinsic and intrinsic factors are twined in an endless push-and-pull interaction. We can control extrinsic factors, such as our exposure to sun, wind, cold, cigarettes, and stress. But until now, we could not control the way our DNA responded to those factors, so that even the most diligent sunscreen user could still look old once her DNA ran through its program.

Dermatologists used to believe that the skin's aging was the inevitable result of the abuse women heaped on their skin back when they were carefree teenagers and young adults. Things like baking in the sun with nothing more than baby oil for sun protection or the fun nights spent drinking and smoking and going to bed in the wee hours. As these young women grew older, they'd start to notice some visible (and visibly aging) changes in their skin, and off they'd run to the cosmetics counters for help. But the solutions offered by old-school skin-care products, the endless array of skin peelers and puffers, are only temporary, stop-gap measures. While they do give the skin a few good days of looking bright and buoyant, they ultimately fail to do anything substantial to the underlying damage. What's worse, they leave the topmost layer of the skin even more vulnerable to sun exposure and internal stress.

The reason for this ultimate failure is simple: this kind of skin-care product does not address the skin's interconnectedness—the relationships between the cells and the multiple layers of the skin and the ways in which the skin interacts with the body inside. This kind of product has been designed only to deal with external, extrinsic factors.

Once women realized their medicine cabinet full of products didn't meet their expectations for visible changes in their skin, they'd pay a visit to their dermatologists for help. And they would get help, with the products that came in the first wave of the New Skin-Care Revolution: treatments like alpha-hydroxy acids (AHAs), chemical peels, injectable fillers that replace lost volume, microdermabrasion, and lasers. These treatments provided genuine short-term solutions, clearing out dead layers of skin, stimulating collagen and blood flow, replacing lost volume, and making skin glow.

But these results didn't last either. They couldn't. They hadn't been designed to *reprogram* the skin from the inside out.

What *can* reprogram skin are compounds that turn on collagen production so that skin thinks it's a teenager again (without the acne, thank you!) while turning off the collagen-destroying enzymes of old age. We now have ingredients that strip away old, dead skin and rebuild it with fresh cells. We now have enzymes that cleanse damage from DNA and restart it on a new path of skin building.

This has happened because our fundamental understanding of intrinsic aging has changed completely. We now understand that the aging clock starts ticking when the instructions run out and speeds up due to an accumulation of unrepaired damage to DNA. Each new nick to the DNA strand weakens it ever so slightly, until the burden of breaks leaves the DNA and its instructions unusable. In other words, intrinsic aging is caused by the DNA instructions expiring, overlaid on a bed of cumulative damage.

If, however, you can *repair* the DNA and stop the strands from weakening and breaking, you can combat this slow ticking. When you stop the DNA from expiring—and *reprogram* it to switch back on—you can restart its fundamental function. Once that happens, you'll find yourself with skin that regenerates itself naturally, the way it did when you were young.

This is the essence of the New Skin-Care Revolution: undoing intrinsic aging itself!

In the chapters in part 3, I'll explain in greater detail about how discoveries made by molecular biologists—in the form of vitamins, amino acids, and enzymes—can reset the DNA clock, restoring youthful vitality to skin. There is a growing arsenal of new ingredients with as-yet-unfamiliar names, such as endonuclease, ergothioneine, ursolic acid, and niacinamide, that can fine-tune the skin's inner workings—its very metabolism, in fact—in order to protect, energize, and reinvigorate the skin for years to come.

In chapters 13 and 14, you'll find lists of specific products and suggested regimens that can literally reprogram your skin.

Bottom line: The New Skin-Care Revolution is about changing skin for the long haul by tuning up the way DNA controls the skin aging process.

PART II

■　　■　　■　　■　　■　　■

PACKAGING
AND
INGREDIENTS

■　■　■

TWO

Cutting Through the Hype

Hype sells.

When it comes to cosmetics, hype sells very well indeed. Who wouldn't want skin like Uma Thurman or Queen Latifah as it appears in the plentiful ads in women's magazines—glowing and unlined, without a pimple, crease, or freckle in sight? The desire is even sharper today because women feel younger than their calendar years, and they want to look as good as they feel.

Yes, hype sells hope.

Anyone who loves cosmetics and wants to look younger needs only to walk into Sephora or the beauty aisles in a large department store to be transported into a literal Garden of Eden of skin-care delights. Row after row of products, in shiny boxes and sleek round jars, trumpeting claims that verge on the near-miraculous. Alongside the new species of high-tech products with ingredients you've never heard of (and can barely pronounce) are stacked the tried-and-true brands from famous names, lined up near the all-natural organic lines and the classic brand your aunt Doris swears is still the best.

Yet many of these gorgeously packaged and cleverly promoted products—you know, the one that just splashed the seductive two-page spread in *Allure,* or the one that has a waiting list five months long even though it costs a cool thousand bucks, or the other one that is made from the delicate coral so rare that it can only be plucked by specially trained native divers off the coast of an exotic Pacific island—are nothing more than a bedtime story. There is no proof for their claims, even if the salespeople swear they're for real. In fact, many studies by respected scientists published in medical journals directly debunk these false promises.

So how can you tell what works? And not just works—but works for *you*?

It's probably true that because hype sells so well to those who are anxious for *some* kind of skin-care product to work—*anything*, in fact—most cosmetics companies don't actually have to tell the customer if there is any science behind the miraculous claims. That's not great news for consumers, as it means that solid and understandable information about the effectiveness of these products is tough to find.

I know that good products are out there. But figuring out which skin-care products you need and which ones you don't is not easy. Armed with the right tools—in the form of what I'm going to tell you in the next two chapters and throughout the rest of the book—you will soon be able to saunter into any cosmetic aisle and waltz out again with skin-care products that will actually make your skin look better.

Without an overstuffed shopping bag—and without breaking the bank.

ALL YOU REALLY NEED

A good skin-care regimen includes a serious dose of prevention, no matter what your age, along with the latest technology to reverse past damage. I'll go into much greater detail about these specific ingredients and concepts in part 3, but let's start with the basics of what you need to look for in over-the-counter (OTC) products.

SKIN-CARE CATEGORIES

The heart of a treatment product is not its evocative name, its come-hither ads, or the fact that even though it's incredibly expensive it was sold out the day it hit the market. What really matters are the benefits it delivers.

Despite the wide array of products available, they actually fall into only six categories, making only a few distinct claims. These are

- Sun protection or recovery from sun exposure
- Moisturization
- Anti-irritation
- Anti-aging, antiwrinkle
- Exfoliation
- Lightening (bleaching) or darkening (tanning) the skin

Within these categories, here's what to look for—and to avoid:

What Works
Alpha-, beta- and polyhydroxy acids and peels
DNA repair
Multitasking formulas with several active ingredients
Solutions that treat several integrated functions of the skin at
    once
Vitamin A and retinol
Vitamin C
Vitamin E

What's Overrated
Antioxidants
Peptides
Products with only "natural" ingredients
Products with only botanical extracts
Products with one "miraculous" ingredient
Super cleansing, with antimicrobials
Tanning for sun protection
UVA radiation

What's Underrated
Active ingredients purified from plants
Common sense
Lipids for moisturizing
The effects of genes and family history on skin
The effects of nerves and emotions on skin
The effects of the immune system on skin

While the ingredients themselves are key (and I'll cover this in more detail in chapter 3), *how many* products you need is important, too. The success of a good skin-care routine isn't measured by how many products are used or how many steps there are. When it comes to skin care, less is often more.

The best new products currently available have been designed to address multiple needs simultaneously. They're multitaskers. A well-designed treatment product doesn't have one "miraculous" ingredient. Instead, it combines all the active agents necessary for its specific role in your skin-care regimen, whether as sun protection, moisturizing, or exfoliation. (So, for example, you might be interested in a product that claims to help fight aging because it exfoliates and contains both antioxidants and anti-irritants.)

Fewer products mean you're more likely to actually use them and actually gain their benefits. Fewer products means you'll be able to observe clearly what works best on your particular face and what doesn't. Fewer products also means fewer opportunities for irritation or other reactions to develop. And, of course, fewer products mean you'll be saving hundreds of dollars every year on products that you don't really need.

If you follow the right, well-thought-out regimen, you'll only need one or two multitasking products along with a sunscreen in the morning and a cleanser and one or two products at night. Add to this an occasional exfoliation and attention to specific problems, and that's it. The only exception is if there are chronic conditions such as acne or hyperpigmentation (age) spots that require longer and more substantial treatment.

So now that you know how little you really do need, let's tackle the monster under the beauty bed: cosmetic hype.

WHAT ARE COSMETICS AND COSMECEUTICALS ANYWAY?

COSMETICS

Let's start with the basics: the definition of "cosmetics," which for seventy years has governed the way in which products and product information have been presented to us—and, in turn, the way we view the prospects for improving and rejuvenating our skin.

It all started with the basic distinction between a cosmetic and a drug, which was marked with the passage of the Federal Food, Drug, and Cosmetic Act of 1938. (To put it in perspective, that was the year that Bette Davis won her second Oscar!)

As defined by the act, cosmetics are products "for cleansing, beautifying, promoting attractiveness, or altering the appearance." This category covers all OTC products readily available without a prescription. Prescription drugs, on the other hand, are defined by the FDA as products that can *change* the structure and function of skin. Drugs must all pass stringent testing requirements to receive FDA approval.

The Food, Drug, and Cosmetic Act had positive effects. It made skin-care products safer, for one thing. And it also established a single federal standard for skin-care products—thereby avoiding individual standards for each of the then forty-eight states. But science has since catapulted well beyond the arbitrary cosmetic/drug division made in 1938. Today, that distinction has been blurred if not entirely erased.

Take, for example, one of the most widely used ingredients of all: water. Sensitive laboratory instruments can measure changes in the structure and function of skin after a cotton ball soaked in water has been applied to it. Of course, plain old water is not a drug! But much more to the point, today, at any department store, beauty boutique, or drugstore, we can purchase a dizzying array of treatment products containing ingredients that are by no means considered drugs, but that really do repair, restore, and rejuvenate. Most moisturizers, toners, AHA creams, as well as those containing vitamins A, C, and E, demonstrably change the structure and functioning of skin. These ingredients are not drugs—they just *act* like them. Or at least they do according to the Food, Drug, and Cosmetic Act of 1938!

The notion that skin-care products can so easily be relegated to separate categories is now considered old-fashioned and quaint—a part of cosmetics history. Yet this legal distinction continues when it comes to product labeling and descriptions in ads and promotional materials. In order to remain in complaince with the law, today's cosmetics market follows a more practical definition.

In other words, products are classified as cosmetics based not on what they actually do, but by what is said about them. Cosmetics aren't legally allowed to change the skin—they can only help consumers look and feel better. Therefore manufacturers can't say they alter the skin, even if they do. The emphasis on "improving how the skin appears" is paramount.

Is this really good for consumers? Hardly. Other countries, like Japan, have more up-to-date product categories and stringent standards. But until Congress passes a new cosmetic act to bring the skin-care world into the twenty-first century, consumers will continue to be bombarded by fuzzy claims and confusing advertising.

Bottom line: The legal straitjacket put on what can be said about cosmetics means that they are promoted with carefully crafted but baffling advertising.

COSMECEUTICALS

Back in the late 1980s, the first wave of the New Skin-Care Revolution was heralded by an exciting buzzword: "cosmeceuticals."

The word itself was a clever melding of "cosmetics" and "pharmaceuticals." What it signaled was a new breed of skin-care products engineered not just to color and cover up skin, but to bring an organic change, even if it lasted only for a few hours or a day or two. The implication was that these products worked better than plain old cosmetics but weren't potent enough to warrant FDA scrutiny and prescription status.

Cosmeceuticals started out as the first serious collaboration between researchers, dermatologists, and cosmetic companies to make products that not only felt great but had a real benefit for skin. Products with vitamins A, C, and alpha-hydroxy acids led the way in supporting their claims with clinical proof published in medical journals, and consumers saw their effects right away. These products set a standard for performance that continues to this day.

Soon, though, the very word "cosmeceuticals" became prey to the same hyperbole and overstatement that plagued the older generation of cosmetics. Nearly every new product claimed to be a cosmeceutical and was dressed in pseudoscientific nonsense complete with seemingly magical, if fuzzy, promises. That's because no matter how many wrinkles they remove or how much collagen production they stimulate, cosmeceuticals are still bound by the same advertising rules that govern old-fashioned cold cream or rosewater toner.

In order to stay in compliance with the law, cosmetics companies skillfully manipulate words and phrases to keep FDA lawyers away (and consumers baffled). And so we have ads carefully stating that a product "helps" the skin improve itself—since a product is not officially sanctioned to accomplish that goal on its own.

Once again, is this really good for consumers? Of course not.

See the section on advertising claims in this chapter for more information about what advertising hype to avoid.

Bottom line: Cosmeceuticals are nothing special—just more cosmetics hype.

BRAND LOYALTY

Many cosmetic companies sell a staggeringly long line of products, presenting them as synergistically created regimens. This is smart marketing, as it encourages the consumer to believe that if she doesn't use every item in the line, she'll lose out on potential benefits.

Brand loyalty has its pleasures, of course. It makes for quick and easy purchasing decisions, and if the texture of your favorite brand's moisturizer suits you, you may very well like the skin brightener and the eye cream, too. In fact, all the products in a skin-care line often have a similar base and texture, and it could be that this particular combination suits your complexion. If so, use your common sense, consider yourself lucky, and be as loyal as you like!

With so many new ingredients and technologies available today, it's a smart idea to select new products carefully and rotate them into your routine. Be sure to try only one new product at a time—that way, if you develop a reaction, the cause will be clear. Be patient. You can't undo a lifetime of skin damage overnight. You absolutely *must* give a new product at least six to eight weeks to prove itself and see if it makes a difference to your skin.

Bear in mind, though, that skin-care products have to be right for you. No one product, even the most popular, can possibly serve everyone—what works on your best friend or even your sister might not be successful for your skin type. It is impossible to know what will work for you without trying it, so always test a product in a store—but only if it comes in a pump. Open testers can be teeming with bacteria.

Never be too shy to ask for free samples of items you are interested in. A great many skin-care products are now so expensive that responsible manufacturers *should* offer samples, to encourage you to try (and also because they know consumers favor companies with generous freebies). While samples usually only contain enough product for a few days' testing, you can still get a good idea if you like the fragrance and texture and see if you have any adverse reactions, such as irritation, itchiness, or rashes.

Bottom line: Look past the brand name to the ingredients and test them out.

THE HARD SELL AT THE STORE

Today, one of the few places to get information about the ingredients in cosmetics is from the people selling them to you, whether at the department store counter in Macy's, a specialty store like Sephora, the kiosk at the mall, or even from the neighborhood Amway representative. There, the sales force is entreating, cajoling, flattering, and gushing, all with two purposes—to get you to buy, buy, buy, and then get you to remain loyal to the brand (or to them), so you keep buying, buying, buying!

It takes the stamina of a marathoner and the determination of an army drill sergeant to circumvent the hard sell. The salespeople are highly trained and they are almost uniformly lovely, but they are usually taught to give a pitch, not the proof. If you ask them to back up their claims, listen carefully—they are scripted to be vague, with meaningless statistics, aided by personal stories of clients who just *love* the new line.

These explanations are often all about how the products will benefit your skin, but they sometimes are about a side issue, such as what the ingredient is, where it came from, or how it is made. This is what marketing people call a reason to believe. These "reasons" suggest that you should like the product regardless of whether it actually helps your skin. It's the ride along the way they're selling, not the real end result.

Many of the most common reasons to believe are listed on product boxes or splashed in glossy ads. These are the most common:

- Free-radical protection
- All natural and environmentally friendly
- Exotic and rare ingredients
- Rain forest botanicals

None of these claims has anything to do with the benefits you will see in your skin. It's up to you to determine which (if any) of these secondary reasons are really important to you (such as protecting the environment) and which are distracting fluff (such as a rare ingredient). Remember that you're not buying anything to make a salesperson or a large corporation happy or to impress your friends and neighbors. You're buying because your skin needs help.

Ask, how does it work? Ask, why is this important?

Once you really start listening, it's not hard to distinguish between what a product can do (sun protection or recovery from sun exposure, moisturization, anti-irritation, anti-aging, exfoliation, and lightening or darkening the skin) and the reason to believe (traditional and rare remedy from the Amazon jungle).

Cosmetic packages are also loaded with buzzwords that seem to say something important but may not deliver all that you expect. Some examples:

Brightening. The cosmetic version of the drug term "lightening." Any brightening product is intended to reduce pigmentation and even out skin tone. Computer-aided devices that measure light reflected from skin can actually measure changes in skin tone, but these are *not* required in order to put this claim on the package.

Clinically proven. This term brings to mind white coats and sterile hospital rooms, but all it really means is that the product was tested on people. Since animal testing has all but disappeared, nearly all skin-care products are tested on people, at least to check for irritation. "Proven" is a matter of opinion, and it doesn't tell you anything about the type of proof or how many people were tested.

Dermatologist tested and recommended. As with "clinically proven," this implies a medical study, but in reality all it means is that a dermatologist reviewed the product in some way. Safety testing is often reviewed by a dermatologist, so nearly all products fit this label, and this claim need not specify what type of testing was done. The dermatologist doing the recommending could very well be someone on the company payroll.

Detoxifying. This term plays on the presumption that our skin is somehow poisoned by our modern lifestyle. If this were really true, you should be consulting your physician rather than seeking advice at the cosmetic counter! Throwing around words like "toxins" is a bit of an exaggeration designed to make a product seem like a rehab center in a bottle. It doesn't say what the toxin is, what the danger is, or how much it's being reduced if it is real.

Firming/lifting. As cosmetics compete with dermatology, these terms have come into use to suggest something that's nearly as good as a face-lift or other surgical procedures. A sensation of firming or lifting can be produced in OTC products that include ingredients that do nothing more complicated than contract when they dry on the skin.

Hypoallergenic. This medical-sounding term often refers to a standard test that should be performed on all products to ensure that they don't produce irritation or allergic reactions. The test is called a repeat insult patch test, and it means the product was applied repeatedly over three weeks to the skin of volunteers, who were subsequently examined for redness and rashes.

Noncomedogenic. This term is used on products designed for oily skin or that treat acne, and it means the product does not produce or aggravate acne. It also refers to testing done on people, usually with a dermatologist involved. It doesn't mean that a product *cures* acne, only that it doesn't make it worse. And it doesn't mean that this product won't cause irritation or rashes, either.

Oil free. Because most consumers fear that oil in products translates to oily skin (which it shouldn't), this term plays on that fear by implying that any amount of any oil is bad for skin. In this chemically complex world, though, an "oil" can slip into the product by changing its name to "extract." Most often, the dreaded oils have merely been replaced by silicones.

Bottom line: Ask questions and listen carefully to make sure the answers make sense. Now you can decode some of the buzzwords!

THE MANUFACTURER'S REPUTATION

Almost everyone knows who made their car or handbag, but few pay attention to exactly who makes their cosmetics. The product manufacturer is always listed at the bottom of the back label, and often can be found on the front of the outer packaging. A major brand-name company means that the product is almost certainly safe and pleasing to the touch—yet that is no guarantee that it works.

Be a smart consumer. Realize that large-scale manufacturers may (or may not) spend a lot of money on research, but they also have to satisfy a broad range of customers, and that means they avoid many specialty ingredients that might work for a few but that might prove irritating to some consumers. So they sacrifice effectiveness for ingredients that have broad appeal.

Smaller brands can risk being on the cutting edge, focusing on special needs and competing for attention with advanced technology. They might have made products just right for you, but you are going to have to go out and find them. Then ask for samples so you can test them at home.

Many dermatologists have entered the skin-care market in the last few years, and some have terrific products. Others are good but not worth the markup. Bear in mind, too, that dermatologists selling their own lines may or may not have had a hand in the lines' development. Some buy off-the-shelf products from popular suppliers and simply place a label with their name on it and pass it off as their own. You should never feel pressured to purchase products by your doctor. Listen carefully so you can spot the new products with proven benefits.

The world of skin care can be too tempting even for physicians with no particular expertise. Take Dr. Andrew Weil, the healthy aging guru. He had previously been quite scathing in his assessment of these products in his 2005 book, *Healthy Aging*: "The first thing to be said about [cosmetic] products on today's market . . . is that most of them are bogus . . . in the case of cosmetics, the claims are even sillier, the lack of evidence more complete . . . I am unconvinced that any of the ingredients in these expensive products has anti-aging effects."

Apparently at the time he wrote this he had not yet familiarized himself with the vast amount of scientific and medical literature explaining the very real virtues of sunscreens, DNA repair, AHAs, microdermabrasion, retinoids, vitamin C, and other active ingredients. He clearly changed his mind, because he endorsed a product line called Dr. Andrew Weil for Origins launched in late 2005, featuring Plantidote Mega-Mushroom serum and cream (whatever that is!). If a well-respected physician can be so mixed up about skin care, it's no surprise that consumers are confused!

Bottom line: Consider who is making the product—bigger is not always better. Physicians may know skin medicine, but that doesn't mean they know more than anyone else about making skin products.

PRODUCT POETRY

Although most women can instantly analyze the nutritional contents of a cereal box at the grocery store, they don't know what to look for when they pick up a cosmetics package at the department store counter.

For the most part, cosmetics are packaged in boxes or containers with very little hard-core information appearing anywhere on them. How could they, when most of the space is dedicated to esthetics, leaving just the bare bones of what's legally required by the FDA: simple instructions and a list of ingredients? There's literally no room left (or any desire) to describe the evidence that the product works.

So let's take a look, as we would in the supermarket, at the package itself. With a little practice you will be able to strip this package down to basics to see what the product does, what's in it, and the results you should expect from it.

NAME AND DESCRIPTION

The largest print on the front of the package should state the product brand as well as its name. Some names are short and sweet; some include a string of adjectives, like "Timeless Anti-Aging Complex Preventive Botanical Exfoliating Wrap," that seem to say a lot when they're really not saying much at all! Believe it or not, such names have almost always been carefully selected by marketing experts, whose job it is to set the mood for consumers, convincing you that you absolutely must take this cleanser or toner home.

Nearby, in letters no less than half the size of the product name, is some kind of description, such as "moisturizer," "eye cream," or "exfoliating gel," which should tell you what kind of product it is and/or what it does. Yet the description may be designed to communicate subconsciously that the product is unique, without telling you exactly why. Be wary if you can't understand the description. What exactly is a "revitalizing complex," for instance?

Another important factor to consider is the amount of the product inside the container. Don't rely on how big the container looks. Check the lower end of the package front for the amount—the precise amount is required by law. This is shown as ounces (oz) and often as milliliters (ml). Remember, appearances can be deceiving. Sometimes bottles or jars can have false bottoms, or tubes may be built with inner linings, or boxes are provided that are much larger than necessary. These make the contents look more sizable than the same amount in another container. So when you're comparing products, don't just check the prices, but the number of ounces, too.

Bottom line: Good products clearly state what they are, what they do, and how much of the formulation is in them. Don't be fooled by fancy words and packaging.

HOW A BOX LOOKS

Skin-care companies take great care and spend countless millions devising and designing the packaging that surrounds a product. The intention is not just to make the product and the brand instantly recognizable, but to confer a style, a look, and a sensibility to which the consumer can relate.

The best designers develop what's called a "visual language"—images that cause you immediately to associate the package with happy memories, things you aspire to, and objects of your desire. Some of them are deliberately designed to evoke an old-fashioned apothecary look, while others aim for a no-nonsense, pared-down appearance so that they resemble prescription drugs. Still others go for a sleek, chic look that screams "I'm expensive and luxurious—how about you?"

According to a recent study among European women, the style of packaging does influence how the product is used—in a surprising way. It seems that fancy packaging causes consumers actually to use *less* of the product recommended for each application, as an innate hoarding instinct kicks in to make the presumably expensive cream last longer. As a result, a product in a fancy package is less likely to be used correctly, and thus becomes less effective, than the same product in plain packaging! Remember, once you buy the product, forget about the price— use it the way it's intended to see if it works. Then decide if it's worth it to buy more.

Bottom line: It's okay to enjoy the packaging if you know what you are getting.

INSTRUCTIONS FOR USE

The FDA mandates that all skin-care products have instructions written on the box or the container. (It doesn't say that they should be written in minuscule type, though!) Most often, instructions are found on the back of the container or box, in the second paragraph, leading with the phrase "How to Use," "Directions," or "Instructions." You should be advised whether to apply this product morning or night, once or twice a day. You'll also be informed as to where it goes on the body and sometimes (although it should be always) how much to use.

Before you buy, ask yourself: Will this product fit into my daily regimen, or is it an occasional remedy? How am *I* going to use it?

There are, in fact, no hard and fast rules, and you can try the product anywhere on your body. Just be careful with the skin around your eyes, which is thin and prone to irritation, and you certainly don't want any creams or lotions on your eyeball itself. A face moisturizer can definitely double as a hand balm; a foot cream can do wonders for parched elbows.

Don't, however, use more than is indicated because you think you'll get it to work faster or better. Doubling the right amount of moisturizer will not double its effectiveness. Quite the opposite. The more product you use, the more likely it is to interfere with other products or the skin itself and the more likely you are to see an unwanted reaction to it blossoming on your face.

Bottom line: As with anything else, *read the directions!*

INFORMATION INSERTS

The FDA mandates that a detailed information insert accompany any prescription drug. In very small type on very thin paper, you can read an often incomprehensible (but clinically correct) explanation of what the drug is, how it works, contraindications, and potential side effects.

Detailed inserts with this kind of information are rarely found in skin-care products because they aren't prescription drugs and can't make druglike claims. They're also not widely found because consumers don't demand them. This is really a shame. What *is* widely found is a piece of paper with a small amount of product hype translated into seventeen languages so the same package can be sold around the world.

This is changing, slowly, beginning with products sold in doctors' offices. One sign of those products that are a part of the New Skin-Care Revolution is that they contain informative package inserts designed to help the consumer understand how to gain the benefits touted in the advertising.

Bottom line: Look for products with detailed descriptions of how they work to help you decide if you really want or need them.

CONTAINERS AND HOW THEY WORK

Containers are more than just aesthetic—for a scary reason. The number-one problem with cosmetics is bacterial contamination from skin and air. Preserving cosmetic products from this contamination is a major challenge.

Jars are the worst offenders, since they are designed to be opened and closed frequently, exposing the entire surface of the product to air-borne contaminants, as well as bacteria from the fingers that are dipped into the jar.

Tubes have the familiar problem of push-out and suck-back between the inside and outside of the package.

Pumps are better, but those with long straws leading into the lotion or cream draw the product up from the bottom and still leave air on top of the product.

Airless pump bottles are the best. There, the contents are pushed up from the bottom by a plunger, so no air is trapped inside with the product.

A metered dispenser is another excellent feature that pumps out the same amount every time the plunger is pushed. This feature avoids the waste when too much product is inadvertently squeezed from a tube or dipped from a jar and can make a small pump dispenser last as long as a much bigger tube.

Bottom line: Consider the safety and cleanliness of a package after you open it—airless pumps are best.

AT WHAT PRICE?

Let's be blunt: High price does not mean high quality. This is especially true in recent years, when manufacturers have been competing to produce the most expensive products without regard to whether the ingredients work together in a potently synergistic way—or whether they justify the cost to the consumer.

On the other hand, given production costs (from research and development, raw ingredients, processing, packaging, shipping, marketing, overhead), a low price (under fifteen dollars for 3.4 oz/100 ml) for an active skin-care product, such as an antiwrinkle cream or multitasking moisturizer, means that less than one dollar went into the ingredients. This pretty much guarantees that the product does not take advantage of the newest skin-care technology. But on the other hand, it doesn't mean that the product doesn't do what it says it's going to do!

The average product sells for a stupendously high markup in relation to the cost of the raw ingredients and production overhead. Contrary to claims, there is no one ingredient that is so effective that it warrants any skin-care products being sold for more than three hundred dollars—which is more than nearly all FDA-approved drugs for skin. And some now cost in the *thousands!*

The whole pricing game can really be a selling strategy. You might not be able to afford the $950 top-of-the-line cosmetic, but hey, don't worry, you can get the downsized, slightly less potent little-sister product for a mere $150. Doesn't that sound good? Aren't you worth it?

You certainly won't be told that rare and hard-to-find ingredients used in small amounts don't necessarily do any good to the actual product—they only promote the belief that they're worth the cost. Kanebo Sensai Premier The Cream, for instance, contains a rare Japanese seaweed and sells for $650 a 1.4-ounce bottle, but there is no scientific proof that this seaweed, or any other seaweed, has any special effects other than to puff up the price.

Some companies take the opportunity to "dust" a product, which means to sprinkle a vanishingly small amount of an intriguing ingredient in the formula and then tell the whole story of all of its supposed

---

The "Dusting" of CoQ10

CoQ10 is a highly touted antioxidant, whose patent is owned by QPharma. When QPharma discovered that the Curél Age Defying Therapeutic Moisturizing Lotion was making the claim that it "now contains the natural power of Q10, [which] helps reveal healthier skin," it sued Andrew Jergens, Curél's parent company, for patent infringement.

At issue was the fact that QPharma had never licensed Jergens to use its patented ingredient. In its defense, Jergens argued that it used no more than 0.00005 percent CoQ10 in the Curél product, an amount it acknowledged was too meager to be "effective."

From a legal standpoint, this was proof that Jergens was not using the QPharma patent, and QPharma was forced to drop its case.[1] The biggest loser, though, was the consumer, who may have bought the Curél product rather than another because they believed it had an effective antioxidant in it, when in fact the amount was infinitesimal and ineffective.

benefits. (See "The 'Dusting' of CoQ10.") One way you can spot dusting is to look at the ingredient list and see whether the magic ingredient appears toward the top of the list (present in larger quantities) or near the bottom of the list (making a cameo appearance). You'll learn more about how to read the ingredient list in chapter 3.

Where does the money go for a typical product? Let's consider a high-end anti-aging product you might buy at a chain drugstore, a category the business calls the "mastige" market. (It's a bit of an oxymoron: the fusion of the words "mass" and "prestige." The magic of advertising is that it can make something available on the mass market seem prestigious!)

Let's say the product costs thirty dollars. The first fifteen dollars goes to the store, of which three dollars is kicked back up to the chain headquarters to support the national television advertising and circulars that stuff your mailbox.

That leaves fifteen dollars for the manufacturer. He uses about seven of those dollars for his own advertising campaign in the glossy women's magazines and sexy billboards along the highway. So a total of at least ten dollars (three from the chain and seven from the manufacturer) of the original thirty-dollar price tag goes into trying to convince you to buy the item.

That leaves eight dollars of the original thirty for the product itself. The manufacturer will use four dollars or more of that to buy a nice bottle and put it in a package with perhaps a false bottom, great graphics, and an enchanting name. And for going to all that trouble he needs at least two dollars in profit per jar.

That leaves just about two dollars of the original thirty for *all* the ingredients, including the cream base, the pH adjuster, the emulsifier, the fragrance, and the preservative. If there is anything left over, it just might go into the latest high-technology botanical extract that is the greatest discovery of the century and will completely revitalize your aging looks!

Bottom line: High price and rare ingredients don't prove anything, but low price means a product probably hasn't incorporated new technology.

HOW TO SPOT FALSE CLAIMS

Now that you know that you're not likely to find out too much about a product from its packaging and that it may be like pulling teeth to get it from the sales representative, where can you find answers to the questions you're still likely to have?

Let's take a look at how companies share the love.

ADVERTISING CLAIMS

Beautiful faces are everywhere—in print advertisements, broadcast commercials, streaming videos, Web sites, even cell-phone ads. Although they are restricted from making drug claims, company-controlled messages, whether visual or verbal, are engineered to convey maximum propaganda while at the same time enticing you to buy, use, repeat.

Visual messages are the first ones you process when you look at an ad, and these have traditionally come in two distinct forms. One features the product as an icon, conveying power and authority from within. The other features a woman—sometimes a model, sometimes a celebrity—conveying the hidden message *I am beautiful and desirable. If you choose this product, you'll look just like me.*

Such an aspirational appeal of a brand image is highly enticing. Even though most of us have a pretty good idea that every woman has different skin-care needs, who's to say that we won't look a little bit more like Elizabeth Hurley if we use the creams she's selling? At least we can "feel" like Elizabeth Hurley.

Some cosmetics companies have also wised up to the spending power of the baby boomer and the young old. They've chosen slightly more realistic models and mature celebrities in ads and commercials, such as Catherine Deneuve for M·A·C Cosmetics and Sharon Stone for Christian Dior's Capture Totale anti-aging line.

These examples notwithstanding, you don't have to be a cynic to realize that the average age of a skin-care supermodel is just past puberty and that even the most gorgeous skin has been photoshopped to perfection, whether the model is fifteen or fifty-five.

Verbal messages come in the form of text. Cosmetics ads typically contain only about fifteen words of message, intended not so much to convey factual information as the brand ambiance. Such short (and often deliberately) vague descriptions have gradually acquired an advertising and promotional vocabulary of their own. It's pretty easy to crack the code—just look for certain verbs like "helps" or "fights" or modifiers like "may improve," "may enhance," and "visible difference." You'll read that Product X doesn't rejuvenate the skin by itself, but rather *helps* the skin with self-renewal. Medical terms are forbidden, but related generic terms are acceptable: a "skin lightener" is a drug, but a "skin brightener" is a cosmetic. "Reversing" fine lines and wrinkles takes a drug, but "fighting" them is a job for a cosmetic. These soft and indefinite phrases are required by FDA regulations but create confusion. They make it harder to figure out if the product really does something or just wants to be included in the category without actually working. By recognizing these key words you'll know at least what changes to look for in your skin when you are using it.

In addition, some cosmetics companies spend millions on marketing their products as an OTC alternative to Botox or other skin-rejuvenating procedures performed in dermatology and plastic surgery offices. *Come to us and we can help you,* skin-care companies propose, *instead of getting that filler injection or going under the knife.* And of course, these products are especially enticing for those who are needle phobic or can't afford Botox or fillers, which can be extremely expensive. Yet no OTC product can do what a scalpel does. Nor can cosmetics replace lost volume the way an injectable filler can or erase wrinkles the way Botox can.

Bottom line: Advertising appeals to us with pictures and words, and it's okay to enjoy them! If you're confused by incomprehensible terminology, it's not your fault but rather a giveaway that the product is nothing more than an ambitious hope. Just learn to decode the message and hone in on the details about what's inside the package.

PICTURE PERFECT
Readers love before-and-after photos. They're persuasive proof of visible changes, clear-cut evidence of improvement and diminished wrinkles, right? How can you NOT believe what's staring right back at you?

Quite easily, as a matter of fact.

Before-and-after photos can be biased in many ways. Take a really good look at the photos in an ad next time you see them. Chances are that the conditions were not identical. The subjects tend to look haggard and frowning in the before pictures, with unflattering light and little, if any, makeup. In the after photos, though, *voilà!* Strategic lighting, expert makeup, styled hair, sweet smiles—and let's not forget the magic of computer imaging programs. Since you're shown only the two pictures the seller wants you to see, there's no way a valid comparison can be made.

Dermatologists and plastic surgeons are also fond of the before-and-after photos. Often, their photo books haven't been doctored, the subjects aren't wearing any makeup, and they've tried to make the comparison fair. Sometimes, though, there's more to these photos than meets the eye. Take Mary, a suburban mother of three in her late thirties with a demanding administrative job. She consults with a noted dermatologist, Dr. Lookgood, about the tired appearance that's crept onto her face. Dr. Lookgood invites her to participate in a study for some new products he's promoting. Both the products and the office visits will be free during the study and later made available to Mary and the half dozen other participants at discount prices.

Mary willingly poses for her before photo at Dr. Lookgood's office and then is carefully instructed about how to use the products. She does so conscientiously, more so than she ever did her own cosmetics. She's very much aware of being scrutinized and wants to please her doctor, who has such a wonderful reputation, so she takes especially good care of herself.

Two months later, the study is completed, and Mary's after picture is taken. Mary is thrilled to see a visible improvement in her skin. The before Mary was tired and discouraged, her skin neglected. The after Mary is upbeat, having achieved a goal and earned praise from a well-respected medical professional.

The point here is that the difference in the two photos may have nothing to do with the product. Mary carefully attended to her skin for months, and the results showed. What Mary didn't know is that almost any product will produce an improved condition when a woman's skin is pampered and carefully coddled.

Medicine has long recognized that simply paying attention to your health, regardless of the drug or treatment, almost always produces an improvement. This is called the "placebo effect" and explains why valid studies compare the test product with a placebo. The two groups are treated identically, except that one receives the product and the other receives a placebo; neither knows which.

The placebo effect is one of the main reasons that before-and-after pictures are of dubious value.

Bottom line: Before-and-after pictures are not the best proof that a product works.

SCIENTIFIC CLAIMS

Whether products state that they'll fix your skin today or prevent changes in the future, the better ones support their claims with scientific, lab-tested evidence. Here are some of the ways studies are presented to consumers.

Pseudoscientific Studies

Among prestige brands, a race has developed to see who can claim visible effects in the shortest time. First it was two weeks, then two days, then overnight, and now we're down to instantaneously.

All too often, however, in order to satisfy these competitive demands, product claims reach too far and become misleading. One common tactic is the pseudoscientific study, which usually makes use of statistics and must be read carefully.

A typical pseudoscientific study will say something like "76 percent improvement in wrinkles," implying that one can expect three-quarters of facial wrinkles to disappear. But upon closer inspection, the study asked participants whether they noticed any difference, and 76 percent said yes. You don't have to be good at math to realize that the fact that 76 percent of a group liked the product is *not* the same as a 76 percent improvement. It could have simply been a 1 percent improvement noticed by 76 percent of the panelists.

And when you add that participants in studies naturally want to please those who are paying them, these types of studies quickly lose their persuasive appeal.

Doctors' Patient Studies

Another common type of study often cited by the doctor-driven brands is one in which the products are tested by physicians on their patients. This conjures up the image of a physician carefully mixing a custom-designed elixir with a mortar and a pestle in his stark white clinic and doling it out to his devoted and fortunate patients.

Typically, however, the formulas being tested have been produced by a contract lab that is independent of the doctor's office. Unfortunately, these types of studies are biased by the understandable desire of most patients to please their doctor by reporting positive results and by the equally understandable desire of doctors only to see and report the results that confirm their preconceived ideas.

Double-Blind, Placebo-Controlled Studies

The most reliable clinical testing today is the double-blind, placebo-controlled study. With this kind of study, the physician doesn't know whether the medication he is giving his subjects is the active drug or an inactive placebo. The patient obviously doesn't know either, which is what makes it "double blind."

Double-blind studies ensure that the results are not biased by doctors and patients meeting each other's expectations. In many such studies, the group using the placebo actually gets better—yes, it's the placebo effect again!

Double-blind studies are expensive to perform and monitor rigorously because many subjects are needed for the statistics to be meaningful, and half of them don't even get the active product. The studies often stretch out over many months, if not years. Any physician who has performed a double-blind study on a product is certainly going to say so. So it's a fair assumption that if it's *not* mentioned on the box, in the advertisement, or on the Web site, the study in question was likely not double-blind or carefully controlled.

The Side-by-Side Study

One effective measure, less widely used than it should be, is the side-by-side study. It avoids many of the difficulties of the double-blind study. Here, the product and placebo are applied in proximity to each other on the skin—for example, on the left and right side of the face (sometimes called a "split-face" study) or on two spots on the arm or buttocks. In such cases, the active agent and placebo can be compared directly at the same time in the same person, which narrows the chance for bias. In fact, this is the study design for determining SPF ratings in sunscreens, and it's been approved by the FDA since 1975.

Association with Universities

Cosmetic companies have turned to associations with well-respected universities to lend credence to their marketing claims. Research centers, always in need of funding for scientists, have cautiously accepted their overtures. The first was the Shiseido Company of Japan, which in 1989 established the Cutaneous Biology Research Center, affiliated with Massachusetts General Hospital and the Harvard Medical School. In 2005 Clinique Laboratories, a division of Estée Lauder Companies, funded the Clinique Skin Wellness Center in the Department of Dermatology at Weill Cornell Medical College in New York City. It opened a clinic to provide skin-care advice, and a place where Clinique representatives could meet with patients, in 2007.

This process stepped over the line, however, when Cosmedicine, at the time a brand of Klinger Advanced Aesthetics, made an alliance in 2005 with Johns Hopkins University in Baltimore—one that included giving the school shares of stock in the company and prominently displaying the Hopkins name in Cosmedicine advertising. After the agreement came to light in *The Wall Street Journal* in April 2006, the president of the university withdrew from the agreement and required that all references to Johns Hopkins be removed from the company literature. It remains to be seen whether other cosmetic companies can find ways to fund research, and research universities can acknowledge the contribution, without compromising their independence and credibility.

Bottom line: Clinical studies, even by doctors and universities, can have conscious or unconscious biases. In the best studies the product is compared to a placebo. Read the percentages in the advertising carefully to see if it is a percent improvement in a skin problem or a percent of the people using it noticing a difference (however small).

BEAUTY AND THE MEDIA BEAST

Detailed information and scientific reporting about new products are often found in the editorial pages of beauty and fashion magazines, which are widely read by information-hungry consumers. According to a recent survey, nearly 40 percent of women get the majority of their beauty advice from magazines. Writers and editors for these journals are lavished with cosmetic and beauty-product samples, wined and dined at product launch receptions, and stuffed with pages of descriptions and data sheets.

Whatever the size or nature of the media write-up, it tends to be upbeat and noncritical, regarding each new product or treatment with democratic enthusiasm. Rather than provide much-needed unbiased evaluation, the reports most often repeat the marketing slogans and simple explanations spoon-fed by the manufacturers in their press releases.

The reason for this is simple: In most cases, magazines are hamstrung by their dependence on their advertisers. Without these ads, they'd quickly lose their primary source of income and have to shut down. So there's a delicate dance between editors and advertisers, resulting in articles that often avoid probing questions, investigations into spurious claims, or negative comments.

Beauty magazines should recognize that they have an audience hungry for critical information and product evaluation and should serve them meaty articles instead of fluff, puff, and filler. But as long as the need for ads remains, don't look for that to happen.

As for the coverage of skin care on television, well, it not only perpetuates the magazine-type nonjudgmental product presentation; it has turned it into an art form. The success of extreme makeover shows and their cosmetic treatment segments (which *always* show dramatic results) underscores the public's fascination with skin improvement—but it's tinted through rose-colored glasses. Every TV makeover ends in such wild success that it sets up the consumer for disappointment.

Most disappointing are the cosmetic companies' Web sites. Even large companies with animated graphics somehow have no room to list product ingredients, explain what they do, or provide the resources to look up the studies that support the company's claims. Part of the reason is that they don't want to disclose information that might assist a competitor, which is certainly understandable. These products are rarely patent protected, after all, and the cosmetic world is filled with knockoffs.

Another reason is that cosmetics companies don't think that consumers are capable of understanding the science. Since you're reading this book, you obviously know that's not true. *During my time spent with cosmetic customers, companies, and media, I became convinced that the public's knowledge and ability to learn are grossly underestimated by our industry.* This misguided perception runs counter to what we know about women in the marketplace. Women surf the Internet. They use search engines, they do research, they ask questions, they talk to one another and compare notes, and with the right information, they can form their own opinions. They spend money and they deserve to know what they're spending their money on.

For products created in the New Skin-Care Revolution, many of the techniques and ingredients are still unfamiliar, with strange names like "biomimesis," "ceramides," or "isoflavones." Although some companies put information about these new breakthroughs on an insert, most don't. Their rationale is that the explanation for how the product works is quite technical and requires more elaboration than room allows— which I think is bunk!

It's time to stop treating cosmetics consumers as naïve, uninformed women blindly buying the next jar of cream just because the advertising claims it was created by Ponce de León himself. But until these consumers speak up and demand the information they need from the sellers and the beauty media, it's not going to be handed to them.

Bottom line: Consumers understand more than they are given credit for. They can move all companies to provide more information by favoring products, magazines, Web sites, and TV shows that give it to them.

Advertorials

An advertorial is a paid advertisement designed to look like the straightforward text of an article. Advertorials are practically everywhere in the media, appearing in a wide variety of publications from magazines like *Vanity Fair* to newspapers like *The New York Times.*

Advertorials aren't necessarily bad. They can serve an honorable purpose by providing substantial space for a cosmetics company to provide and explain the evidence supporting its product's virtues. But (and this is a big but!) all too often, advertorials make use of writing styles as well as fonts and page layouts that are almost indistinguishable from the publication's editorial content. Many readers don't distinguish between these advertisements and the rest of the magazine's articles or spot the small, much fainter type at the top or the bottom of the pages that must state "Advertisement." There in the small type, you may also see "Special Advertising Supplement" or "Did not involve the reporting or writing of staff."

Advertorials masquerading as articles are also quite prevalent on the Internet, so pay attention if you're researching products online.

An infomercial is akin to an advertorial, except it appears on television and gives consumers an opportunity to instantly buy what's being pitched. The skin-care products that are sold on infomercials with legitimate research backing their claims have a great opportunity to explain their results to their customers. More often, of course, the products are sold on high-pressure hype. So, just because you see a product extolled on television doesn't make the claims true. Be aware that the celebrities (and noncelebrities) endorsing what's being pitched on infomercials have been paid to gush!

THREE

Your Ingredient Glossary

A savvy grocery shopper picking up a box of cereal can look at the list of ingredients, quickly scan for calories and carbs, see whether or not there's high-fructose corn syrup or if the sodium content is too high, and promptly decide if that food is going to end up in her shopping cart—or not.

It's not that easy with skin-care products.

There on the shelves are the New Skin-Care Revolution treatments, stacked alongside the creams with skin-sloughing alpha-hydroxy acids and retinols and the green tea, grapeseed, and pomegranate antioxidants; next to the licorice-based skin lighteners that were so popular in the 1990s; underneath the well-known, cheap, and cheerful brands, those hope-in-a-bottle mainstays containing glycerin, shea butter, seaweed, and collagen in cream form; and around the corner from the exotic (and exotically priced) treatments, whether with crushed pearls, caviar, glacial waters, Brittany seaweed, or some ingredient you've never heard of before.

What do all these ingredients do? Why are they there? Why are so many chemicals with unpronounceable names listed?

The Cosmetic, Toiletry, and Fragrance Association (a private voluntary organization of leading cosmetic companies) mandates that all ingredients be registered with them, their names standardized and listed in a particular way on a product's box. Becoming cosmetics literate means you'll be able to identify precisely what is on this list and figure out what makes each product work. It also means you won't blindly accept the claims made by cosmetics companies, because you'll be able to decipher the complicated names, so you'll know if they're active ingredients, preservatives, or truly essential to the efficacy of the product. You'll also be able to zone in on the precise ingredient that is best suited to your needs. If, for example, you need a rich, emollient, cold-weather moisturizer, you don't need to waste your money on a product intended to lighten the age spots on your hands or firm up your face.

HOW TO READ AN INGREDIENT LABEL

By law, ingredients must be listed in descending order of their percentage, from the highest to the lowest. If an active ingredient is the last one listed, you can make a pretty good assumption that it's there in minuscule quantities.

▪ The very first ingredient is frequently water. It's often identified as "aqua."

▪ Next come the ingredients that give a product its texture. They reduce runniness and provide thickening. Look for words that end in
-one: silicone, adding smoothness and slip
-ane: long carbon chains, sometimes mixed with silicone, for thickening
-ide or -ate: small molecules that thicken water
-pol or -mer: long-chained polymers that solidify a formula.

▪ Active ingredients are used in much smaller concentrations than those that make up the formula's texture, so they are usually listed in the second half of the list. If an ingredient you are interested in is in the last third of the list, its strength is probably low. That may be okay for an active element that is extremely potent, but not for an antioxidant or a moisturizing compound.

▪ Some active ingredients are classified as drugs, even though they are available over the counter. This includes the ingredients in sunscreens. Any ingredients that are drugs must be listed in a separate section labeled "Active ingredients." The other ingredients will then follow in another section labeled "Inactive ingredients."

What's confusing about this is that "inactive ingredients" actually are active—they're just not drugs!

■ Some well-known ingredients are listed with the unfamiliar names of their derivatives, appearing here in descending order of their strength:

Vitamin A: retinal, retinol, retinyl palmitate

Vitamin C: ascorbic acid, ascorbate, magnesium ascorbyl phosphate, ascorbyl palmitate

Vitamin E: tocopherol or alpha-tocopherol, tocopherol acetate.

■ Preservatives, coloring agents, and fragrances are most likely to be found near the end of the list.

A Typical Ingredient List

Take a look at this ingredient list from Olay Complete Plus Ultra Rich Moisture Lotion. The explanation of what each ingredient does is listed on the right.

Active ingredients	
6.0% octinoxate	Sunscreens (Sunscreens are required by FDA to be separated from cosmetic ingredients because they are considered drugs.)
3.0% zinc oxide	

Also contains a special blend of: (these are the "inactive" ingredients)	
Water, glycerin	At the top of the list, these are present in the highest concentration and serve as the base lotion
Isohexadecane	Long-chained chemical thickener
Polyacrylamide	A gelling agent
C13–14 isoparaffin	Waxy thickener
Laureth-7	Detergent to make all the ingredients mix together

Cyclopentasiloxane	Silicone for smoothness
PEG/PPG-20/20 Dimethicone	Silicone for smoothness
Steareth-21	Organic chemical to help oil and water mix
Stearyl alcohol	Organic chemical for smoothness
Tocopherol acetate	Vitamin E
Sucrose polycottonseedate	Emollient and skin conditioner
Niacinamide	Vitamin B_3
Fragrance	Chemicals used for fragrance are not re-quired to be individually disclosed
Biphenyl alcohol, cetyl alcohol	Emollient and skin conditioners
DMD Hydantoin	Preservative that releases formaldehyde
Iodopropynyl butyl-carbamate	Preservative
Steareth-2	Organic chemical for smoothness
DEA Oleth-3 phosphate	Organic chemical for smoothness
Panthenol	Provitamin B_5 (must be converted by the body into vitamin B_5)
Disodium EDTA	Preservative
Ascorbic acid	Vitamin C
Vegetable oil	Oil for smoothness
Beta-carotene	Provitamin A (must be converted by the body into vitamin A)
FD&C, Red #4	Dyes to make the formula the right color

This product claims to be a moisture-rich lotion, and the ingredients bear that out. At the top of the list are water and glycerin (a great humectant), and farther down are sucrose polycottonseedate, biphenyl alcohol, and cetyl alcohol to retain moisture. To give the lotion some healthy activity, it's stacked with vitamins A, B_3, B_5, and E, but the first four are well down on the ingredient list, so their effects may be minimal. And to make it a multitasker, it contains two sunscreens (octinoxate and zinc oxide) that give it SPF 15 with broad-spectrum coverage.

As I only had to pay $7.59, I'd say as a moisturizer it is definitely a good buy and well worth it.

Bottom line: You don't need a chemistry degree to recognize the most common skin-care product ingredients. Use this section to analyze your own products to see what you are getting.

INGREDIENTS TO LOOK FOR

These lists of the most common ingredients in skin-care products are listed alphabetically by their purpose. Multitasking ingredients, like vitamin C and ergothioneine, will appear on multiple lists.

ANTIOXIDANTS

Antioxidants are widely used in cosmetics, and we'll take a close look at the proof that they work in chapter 9. There are far too many to list comprehensively, and more are being added every day. But these are the most common antioxidants, grouped by the evidence that they have any benefit at all:

Supporting evidence
Ergothioneine
Genistein
Green tea (or ECGC)
Vitamin C
Vitamin E

Insufficient Evidence — or Don't Believe the Hype
Alpha-lipoic acid
CoQ10
Idebenone
Resveratrol
Soy isoflavones

CALMING INGREDIENTS

These are especially important for use after exfoliation.
Aloe vera
Bisabolol

Chamomile extract

Evodia extract

CLEANSERS

There are hundreds of soaps, nonsoap detergents, emulsifiers, and cleansing agents. These names may seem complicated, but they all are basically the same thing: cleansers!

Alpha-olefin sulfonate

Ammonium lauryl sulfate

Disodium cocoamphodiacetate

Disodium oleamido MEA sulfosuccinate

Polysorbate

Silicone

Sodium cocoyl isethionate

Sodium dodecylbenzene sulfonate

Sodium ether sulfate

Sodium lauryl sarcosinate

Sodium lauryl sulfate

TEA lauryl sulfate

EXFOLIANTS

Alpha-hydroxy acids (AHAs)

AHAs are used at 10 percent or less in OTC products. Check the packaging, labeling, or insert carefully for the pH (acidity). They must be acidic (with a pH less than 5) to work, but bear in mind that a pH lower than 3.5 is irritating.

Alpha-hydroxyoctanoic acid

Glycolic acid

Hydroxycaprylic acid

Lactic acid

Malic acid

Sugar cane extract

Triple fruit acid

Beta-hydroxy acids (BHAs)

These are used only in levels of 1.5 to 2 percent. They also must be in acidic formulas (pH less than 5) to work effectively.

Beta-hydroxybutanoic acid

Salicylic acid

Trethocanic acid

Tropic acid

Polyhydroxy acids (PHAs)

These can be used at up to 15 percent but must also be in an acidic formula (pH less than 5).

Gluconolactone

Lactobionic acid

HYPERPIGMENTATION (BROWN SPOT) FIGHTERS

All these ingredients must be used over several weeks to see an effect. Some, like azelaic acid, kojic acid, and retinol are effective, but high concentrations are needed and they may be irritating.

Arbutin (mulberry extract)

Azelaic acid

Ergothioneine

Kojic acid

Licorice root extract (glycyrrhizinate)

Retinol

Vitamin C

Willow bark extract

MOISTURIZERS

There are hundreds of different moisturizing ingredients and far too many to list comprehensively. Here are some of the most common ones:

Butylene glycol

Cetyl alcohol

Coconut oil

Dimethicone

Glycerin

Jojoba oil

Linoleic acid

Palmitic acid

Petroleum jelly (petrolatum)

Propylene glycol

Safflower oil

Stearic acid

SUNSCREENS

Broad Spectrum — Inorganic

These ingredients are difficult to formulate and leave a white ghosting on the skin unless they're completely rubbed in. They work instantly.

Titanium dioxide

Zinc oxide

Broad Spectrum — Organic

These filter out the broadest range of UV light for high SPF protection. These compounds must be applied at least twenty minutes prior to sun exposure in order to be effective.

Ecamsule (Mexoryl SX)

Helioplex (combination of avobenzone and oxybenzone)

UVA Filters

These filter out the longest wavelengths of light. If used alone, they won't prevent a sunburn, but combined with UVB filters they will provide high levels of protection (see chapter 6). Ingredients that block UVA and UVB are often paired with each other to provide maximum effectiveness and to stabilize each other to prevent them breaking down in sunlight.

Avobenzone (Parsol 1789)

Dioxybenzone

Meradimate

Oxybenzone

Sulisobenzone

UVB Filters

These filter out the shortest wavelengths of light, which are the most damaging to skin. When used alone to achieve an SPF of 15, they inevitably filter out some UVA as well, but to have broad-spectrum protection they must be mixed with one of the UVA filters listed above. They are often used in combination with one another, as some are too weak to work effectively on their own.

Cinoxate

Octisalate

Ensulizole

Homosalate

Octinoxate (octyl methoxycinnamate, Parsol MCX)

Octylcrylene

Trolamine salicylate

TONERS

Toners are supposed to close pores and tighten skin and are discussed in chapter 4. The term has become confusing recently because some manufacturers have labeled true moisturizers as "toners." A real toner has one or more of the following ingredients:

Acetone

Alcohol (ethanol)

Alum

Birch extract

Boric acid

Camphor

Horse chestnut extract

Rosewater

Sandalwood

Witch hazel

WRINKLE FIGHTERS

The market has been flooded with ingredients claiming to treat wrinkles. Here are some of the most widely used, grouped by whether there is evidence to support claims of effectiveness or not.

Supporting Evidence

Alpha-hydroxy acid

Arabidopsis extract

Micrococcus extract

Niacin/niacinamide

Plankton extract

Vitamin A

Vitamin C

Insufficient Evidence, or Don't Believe the Hype

Argireline

Boswelox

Copper peptides

DMAE (dimethylaminoethanol)

Eyeseryl

GABA (gamma-aminobutyric acid)

Matrixyl

TGF-beta

TNS (Tissue Nutrient System) Recovery Complex

Intrinsic Aging Skin Changes and
How to Reprogram Them

The basic premise of the New Skin-Care Revolution has been to identify changes in skin that are programmed by your own DNA. It has also
identified ingredients that can revitalize your skin back to its youthful
functioning. This chart details the genetic changes that take place in aging skin and lists the best ingredients to look for in order to literally reprogram these changes. (Some of these ingredients are so new that they
are not routinely found in products. For more information, take a look
at chapter 10.)

Intrinsic Aging	How It Looks and Feels	Reprogramming	Ingredients to Look For
Outer barrier weakens	Has dry flakes and itches	Increase lipids from inside out	Ursolic acid, licorice extract (glycyrrhetinate)
DNA repair diminishes	Sunburns easily, peels frequently	Supplement DNA repair	Plankton extract, *Micrococcus* lysate, *Arabidopsis* extract
Blood flow lessens	Looks pale, sallow, and feels cold	Stimulate microcirculation	Pinanediol, camphanediol, arginine
Collagen degrades	Shows lines and wrinkles, sags	Increase collagen production, reduce protease digestion	Vitamin C (ascorbic acid), vitamin A (retinol, retinoic acid), ergothioneine
Chronic inflammation persists	Is irritated and itchy	Reduce inflammation, supplement immune system	Evodia extract, bisabolol, Aloeride, *Polypodium leucotomos* (fernblock)

AVOIDING IRRITANTS

Many commonly used ingredients are known irritants. That doesn't mean you'll react to them, and you might react to one in a certain formulation and not in another. If several from this list are found on a product label, it's next to impossible to isolate the specific irritant that affects you. Prior to making a purchase, try to test products on the inside of your arm near your elbow and wait at least twenty-four hours to see if there's any reaction before you buy.

CLEANSERS

These ingredients work well but must be washed off completely in order to avoid any irritation.

Sodium lauryl carboxylate

Sodium or TEA lauryl sulfate

Sulfonates

FRAGRANCES

Fragrances are by far the most common source of irritation. Be aware, though, that "fragrance-free" cosmetics often have an odd smell or use other chemicals in order to mask their natural smell. Fragrances are rarely identified by name.

MOISTURIZERS

These ingredients can be overly drying or trigger other irritation.

Ethanol

Glycerin

Lanolin

Menthol

Methyl nicotinate

Mint

Peppermint

Propylene glycol

Sorbitol

Spotlight on New Ingredients
That Really Do Work

Look for these new ingredients, especially in multitasking formulas.

What It Is	What It Does
Arabidopsis extract	Helps repair DNA
Ergothioneine	Works as an antioxidant, fights hyperpigmentation
Evodia extract	Acts as an anti-inflammatory
Micrococcus lysate	Helps repair DNA
Pinanediol and camphanediol	Increases microcirculation

BOTANICAL EXTRACTS USED IN COSMETICS

Many skin-care products use botanical extracts, many of which do have proven benefits when used in high enough concentrations. Assessing what's good or not can be tricky, though, because the long lists of plant extracts seen on many product labels do not come with an explanation of what precisely those ingredients do. For example, fourteen botanical extracts are cited in the Murad Cellular Replenishing Serum ingredients list, but how can you tell which ones are window dressing and which ones are going to make a difference in your skin?

Here's a list of the most commonly used plant extracts and their intended purpose in skin-care products. Use this list to see if the advertising on the package matches the ingredients in the bottle. I have highlighted in bold letters those ingredients for which there is serious scientific support for their intended purpose. The others are closer to folk medicine. Remember: Just because a product is listed in bold doesn't mean it's there in an effective concentration—you need to check to see how close it is to the start of the list to have an idea if it can work at all. It's hard to pick a product *just* from whether these bold ingredients are in the list, so stick to the recommended products. This information can help you decide what to try, but in the end the real proof is if it works for *you*!

EXTRACT	USE
Aloe vera	Soother; for dry skin and as an aftershave
Arnica	Soother; for healing cuts and bruises
Bayberry	Astringent; used to treat varicose veins
Birch	**Antiseptic, astringent**
Borage	Moisturizer
Broom flowers	Cellulite treatment
Burdock	Antiseptic used for treating acne and eczema
Calendula	**Soother, anti-itch agent; for treating sunburn and wounds**

Camellia sinensis	Emollient, antioxidant
Cat's claw	Antioxidant
Chamomile	**Soother, calmer**
Clary sage	Astringent
Cucumber	Emollient, astringent
Echinacea	Antiseptic; lightener
Fenugreek	Emollient
Fernblock	**Antioxidant**
Ginger	**Soother**
Ginkgo biloba	Antioxidant; targets skin tone and elasticity
Grape seed	**Moisturizer and emollient**
Hops	Toner, skin tightener
Horse chestnut	Astringent; for varicose veins
Jojoba	**Emollient, moisturizer**
Lavender	**Stimulant, invigorator**
Licorice	**Anti-inflammatory, moisturizer**
Macadamia nut oil	**Emollient**
Milk thistle	Antioxidant
Mulberry	**Brightener**
Myrtle	Astringent
Nettle	Astringent; for eczema and sunburn
Papaya	**Exfoliant**
Pomegranate	**Antioxidant, moisturizer**
Red clover	Astringent
Rose oil	Astringent
Sandalwood	**Astringent**
Sesame	Moisturizer
Slippery elm	Emollient for dry skin and as an aftershave
Tea: green, black, or white	**Antioxidant**
White willow	Circulation booster; used to treat acne and eczema
Witch hazel	**Astringent**
Yashabushi	Circulation booster and tightener

Traditional Chinese Medicine for Skin

Many people have the impression that medicine began in Europe and cosmetics were invented in France. In fact, many other cultures have sophisticated potions to treat skin. For example, in traditional, botanical-based Chinese medicine, plant extracts are mixed and melded in what can be considered an art form. According to the precepts of Chinese herbal medicine, a complete elixir has four elements:

- ▓ The king herb, which provides the major benefit
- ▓ The vassal herb, which aids by accentuating the effects of the king herb
- ▓ The assistant herb, which detoxifies any side effects of the king and vassal
- ▓ The servant, which is used to safely transport the king, vassal, and assistant to their site of action.

Take a look at how this principle is translated into a modern product, Boscia Daily Hand Revival Therapy by FANCL of Japan, as described on the side of the package. Each of the elements of traditional Chinese medicine is identified in brackets:

An intensive hand therapy formulated with a powerful antioxidant *Jojoba Leaf* [king herb], and a unique anti-irritant, *Willowherb* [assistant herb], hydrates and revitalizes . . . *Questamide, Wine Yeast, Calendula Flower* [servant herbs] and other conditioning ingredients will nourish . . . *Mulberry* [vassal herb] lightens sun spot pigmentation.

The formula should be effective as a hand moisturizer, although we don't know how much of each extract really appears in the product.

INGREDIENTS FROM FOOD AND PLANT SOURCES

The nutrients from many different foods are often broken down into essences to be used in cosmetics, but they are rarely labeled with their food name. This list will help clear up any confusion. It's also a helpful alert if you have food allergies.

SOURCE	ESSENCE
Carrots	Beta-carotene
Citrus	Ascorbic acid
Cod liver oil	Omega-3 fatty acid
Evodia	Indole quinazoline alkaloid
Fruit acid	Glycolic acid
Grape	Resveratrol
Green tea	Epigallocatechin gallate (ECGC)
Green vegetables	Lutein
Heart and liver	CoQ10, alpha-lipoic acid, idebenone
Milk	Lactic acid
Oats	Avenanthramides
Rosemary	Ursolic acid
Soy	Genistein
Tomato	Lycopene
Vegetable oil	Alpha-tocopherol

ASSESSING THE POTENCY OF THE LISTED INGREDIENTS

How can you assess the potency of different ingredients?

If ingredients are synthesized in a lab, they are either pure or in a mixture (and the manufacturer knows exactly how much of each element is in any mixture). Each batch of product is tested to be sure it meets standards and is consistent. When a synthetic ingredient is used, the formulator specifies what percentage, by weight, should be added to the product. That way we know that each time it's made, the correct amount of a pure substance will be active in a cosmetic product.

When it comes to natural, botanical extracts, however, we don't have that same type of certainty. An extract contains any number of chemical compounds that come out of a plant when it is ground up and soaked in water and alcohol. So we don't know exactly what is in it, and we don't always know what gives the extract its cosmetic benefits. Different manufacturers may even prepare the extract differently. It's a lot like making wine—one batch may be fit for a connoisseur to relish, but another may be more suited for wine that comes in a box.

Wine lovers know that one bottle of Bordeaux can cost ten or a hundred times as much as another. Why is that? Because the variety of grape had a delicate flavor, the soil was better, the rain just right that year, and the vintner harvested the grapes at just the proper moment to produce a heavenly taste.

The same is true of all plants. Flavonoids, alkaloids, and antioxidants—those plant-based active ingredients cherished by the cosmetics industry—vary tremendously by location and climate, just as wine vintages do. Take rosemary extract, pungent and strong. It is used for its soothing and antioxidant properties. But just like the grapes growing in vineyards, the quality of the rosemary plants can vary by the location of the groves from which the leaves are collected, the time of year they were harvested, and the quality of that particular year. How good was the weather? Did it rain at the right time or was there a drought? Rosemary leaves collected from the grove are then sold to a consolidator, who collects from different farms. Then the consolidator sells the leaves to processors, each of whom differ in exactly how they produce each extract. Are the plants ground up in cold water or hot alcohol? Do they soak for a few hours or for several days? Is the final extract filtered once through paper or several times through charcoal? Are preservatives or other chemicals added?

As a result, when our laboratory analyzed five different commercial rosemary extracts, we were not surprised to find that they had widely different compositions. Thus, a name like "extract of rosemary" on a product label is no guarantee that an effective amount is inside the bottle.

Unfortunately, there is no legal requirement that a plant extract contain any particular component in any particular amount. The botanical industry has voluntarily made progress in standardizing extracts; they have set units for many extract components that measure their potency, so two extracts of the same plant from different manufacturers can be compared. The problem is that the potency measures, such as polyphenol content, may not be the reason that the extract is added to the formula, such as to act as an antiwrinkling agent. Bear in mind, too, that a very inexpensive product will be more likely to use a botanical for its name and not its potency.

If you've been using a product based solely on botanical extracts for twelve weeks and have not seen any results whatsoever, I'd say it's fair to assume that the product's potency might be suspect and you should move on to something else with ingredients you can depend on.

Bottom line: The name itself of a favorite botanical ingredient gives you very little to go on when choosing a product, because extracts of the same plant are not equally active. It's still trial and error in choosing botanical products—with lots of errors.

PRESERVATIVES

Preservatives in cosmetics are not to be feared or shunned. Without them, your skin-care product would quickly teem with bacteria and mold that could make you very sick. The number one cause of product recalls in the cosmetic industry is contamination by bacteria.

Preservatives are listed near the bottom of the ingredient list and tend to have long chemical names, often ending in "-ol" or "-ben." There are scores of them used; here is a list of the most common:

Butylparaben
DMD hydantoin
EDTA
Iodopropynyl butylcarbamate
Methylparaben
Phenoxyethanol
Propylparaben
Sorbitol

Whether or not to become preservative free has become a hot-button issue in the skin-care industry. Nevertheless, even as more and more people obsess about germs and carry little bottles of Purell around everywhere they go, the preservative-free movement has somehow managed to convince some consumers that it's healthier not to fight bacte-

Patents

In an effort to avoid disclosing their actual ingredients, products may boast that an ingredient is so secret, *it's patented!*

This is a bit of a sham, as a patented ingredient is anything but secret; it must be publicly disclosed in detail in order for someone to receive a patent on a product. This policy benefits consumers. A patent means that the technology has been written down and has been thoroughly described and that information is freely available. But the mere fact that a patent has been granted does *not* necessarily guarantee that the owner of the patent really invented it. Many patents are struck down when they are challenged in court.

Recently, Dr. Nicholas Perricone and the Medicis Pharmaceutical Corporation became embroiled in a dispute over two of Perricone's patents concerning the benefits of vitamin C on sun-exposed skin. The lawsuit reached the U.S. Court of Appeals,[1] which determined that several sections of Dr. Perricone's patents were not original inventions at all but had already been described by scientists at Chesebrough-Pond's in a patent that had been granted four years earlier.

ria. I can't understand how a mother who rushes to the drugstore for an antibiotic for her child's ear infection can choose a skin-care product because it *doesn't* have an antimicrobial preservative.

Of course, manufacturers are not really willing to give up their major weapon against microbes. They can't—because if they did, their products would quickly become contaminated and unusable. Their solution is to use antibacterial chemicals that are not formally registered as preservatives; in this way, they can still label their products as "preservative free."

Wondering whether or not to go preservative free is also a crucial question when it comes to botanical extracts, such as aloe, soy, lavender, sage, or chamomile, or natural soaps. Extracts can be wonderful additions to skin-care products, but despite all the back-to-nature buzz about them, extracts are by their very nature *not* pure. They are complex mixtures of proteins and sugars, which make a delicious meal for various microbes found everywhere—especially in the air and on our hands. Using unpreserved natural extracts is closer to playing Russian roulette than practicing sound health care.

Bottom line: Steer clear of products that advertise they are "preservative free." Preservatives are a necessary part of skin-care products—don't leave the store without them!

THE ALL-NATURAL FALLACY

Competition among skin-care brands has lately spilled over into claims that their products are socially correct or environmentally friendly, and in theory, that's terrific. The idea is to be natural at all costs, to recycle, to preserve the rain forest, not to use animal testing or preservatives—and still finish with a drop-dead gorgeous look. Yet editors at women's magazines could provide a real service to their readers by taking a closer look at some of these bandwagons before encouraging anyone to jump blindly on board.

The beacon of "all-natural" and "organic" ingredients is a blinding light that will cause many to miss the next phase of the New Skin-Care Revolution. What could sound more enticing than the thought of home remedies taken directly from nature, with sweet-smelling plants lovingly ground into salves to be used as cures for every beauty need? This imagery neglects to include the fact that "all natural" can also mean "all toxic" or "all allergic," or that a skin-care product without preservatives can go rotten before you've even taken it out of the box.

In fact, many of the most potent poisons, like botulinum toxin (found in spoiled food), aflatoxin (rotten peanuts), and psoralen (celery varieties) are all natural. An allergy to peanuts is quite common and can lead to anaphylactic shock and death. Natural ingredients, especially plant oils, are among the most frequent causes of allergic reactions to cosmetics. And how can we forget our favorite all naturals—poison ivy, ragweed, and grass pollen?

Because natural and organic ingredients can be irritating if used in their raw state, cosmetic manufacturers busy touting these extracts neglect to mention how much the ingredients have had to be refined so your skin doesn't turn red and raw after using them. However, in refining the ingredients to remove the irritants, manufacturers often remove the active component! For example, the leaves of the rosemary plant are rich in soothing and skin-building ursolic acid, but commercial rosemary extract is made by grinding the leaves into hot alcohol, collecting the juice, and drying it down to flakes. This removes many of the irritating organic compounds in rosemary leaves, but unfortunately ursolic acid is not very soluble in hot alcohol and is washed down the drain of the factory tanks along with the irritants. As a result, most natural rosemary extract has precious little of one of rosemary's best active ingredients. Look for rosemary extract cosmetic products that highlight ursolic acid, like Remergent Barrier Repair Formula.

Speaking of all natural, the mania over what is *not* in a product has been extended to all cosmetic ingredients derived from animals. This trend began in earnest over concerns about animal testing and gained credibility from the food scare over BSE (bovine spongiform enaphalopathy, or mad cow disease), a brain disease transmitted among cattle and other farm animals that can lead in rare cases to a related disease in humans. Next, *any* ingredient derived from *any* animal was shunned by cosmetic manufacturers—such as the lipids from wool to make cholesterol, eggs to make phospholipids, even fish oils to make emulsifiers. It should be obvious that fish cannot transmit BSE, nor do all animal products require that an animal be killed; just think of wool and eggs. The animal-free mandate has taken several useful ingredients off the market, leaving few substitutes.

"Holistic" is one of the buzzwords of the pure-and-natural movement, but it simply means "taking everything into account." The New Skin-Care Revolution has begun doing exactly that: it considers the integrated systems that control the skin's texture and appearance and looks to nature to find the right match in the right combination to preserve a youthful, vibrant look. By understanding the human genetic code, we better understand how skin is tuned to react to nutrients, weather, and sun. Molecular biology and genetic engineering have been cast as the bad guys, the antithesis of all that's holistic and natural, when in fact they make for ready allies. Nature has spread before us botanicals offering great health benefits, but these active agents often

The Paraben and Phthalate Scares

Not understanding the basic precepts of science can also lead to bouts of temporary hysteria. In 2004, a group of scientists at the University of Reading in the United Kingdom used excruciatingly sensitive equipment to detect trace levels (parts per billion) of the preservative methylparaben in some breast cancer biopsies. The study did not compare the levels in cancer tissue to levels in normal tissue, nor did it determine whether the biopsies came from women who even used methylparaben products.

But since methylparaben is found in deodorants, the news immediately circled the globe that the parabens in deodorants caused breast cancer. Web sites sprang up accusing cosmetic companies of hypocrisy for raising money to fight breast cancer while including parabens in their products. Fearing consumer backlash, major cosmetic manufacturers reformulated their brands, and word went out to suppliers to minimize or eliminate paraben preservatives, even though the European Commission Scientific Committee on Consumer Products reviewed the scientific data in 2005 and concluded that "there is no evidence of a demonstrable risk for the development of breast cancer caused by the use of underarm cosmetics." This episode shows how susceptible consumers are to hype and alleged horror stories. Had the scaremongers carefully examined the original study, I doubt that the ensuing craziness would have occurred.

The problem with phthalates is a little different. Phthalates are used in cosmetics, hair-care products, and nail polish because they contribute a firm but flexible feel. They have been shown to interfere with the normal sexual development of male rats at doses that are 400,000 times greater than the average human exposure. But the publicity storm about phthalates began when a study of two hundred male infants found that those with the least sexual development had the highest levels of phthalates in their urine (presumably from their mothers), although all of the infants were clinically normal. A later study found that the average exposure of a person to phthalates is much lower than the EPA threshhold. No government agency that has reviewed the data has issued a warning. Nevertheless, there may be some risk for women who may become pregnant, so those consumers who wish to be extra careful should check their cosmetic products to be sure they have no phthalates. Most do not.

appear only in tiny amounts and are mixed in with toxins and allergens. The all-natural idea that we must take the good with the bad is a concept that is sorely out of date.

Instead, because of what we now know, we have the tools to select the beneficial essences from the natural world and discard the allergens and toxins. The New Skin-Care Revolution doesn't reject natural. On the contrary, it's all about understanding what is natural on the most fundamental level and harnessing nature to restore the buoyancy and bloom of healthy young skin.

Bottom line: Nature is filled with danger for skin, along with some benefits. "All natural" is not a real advantage but just cosmetic hype. Choose products based on what they do, not what they are.

PART III

■ ■ ■ ■ ■ ■

COSMETIC
PRODUCTS

■　　■　　■

FOUR

Cleansers and Toners

Cleansers and toners are the least glamorous products in the cosmetic cabinet but are the true workhorses of skin care. They must remove not only the dead cells and accumulated dirt on skin, but also the makeup applied each day. For many years they were formulated with simple ingredients that tended to have a drying effect and in some cases left a film that itself had to be removed. But in recent years manufacturers have introduced new ingredients that improved cleaning performance and included additives to jazz the products up for marketing pitches. In this chapter we'll take a look at what characteristics make a cleanser or toner worthwhile.

CLEANSER BASICS

Cleansing is like tending a garden, not like clearing a forest!

The purpose of a cleansing regimen is extremely simple: It should gently remove dirt and cell debris while not stripping the skin of its essential oils and the cell "glue" that holds together the topmost, barrier layer of skin.

Proper cleansing is an essential part of any good skin-care regimen, but squeaky-clean is not the way to go. What you need is the mildest cleanser that will do the job without stripping your skin of essential moisture.

A good cleanser is not harsh. It doesn't leave your skin feeling dry or flaky. It should be composed primarily of mild, water-soluble detergents.

And that's it.

As I explained in chapter 1, the outermost layers of your skin are stacked atop one another like shingles on a roof. This barrier layer, or stratum corneum, is made up of skin cells that die when they reach the surface. They're held together in a kind of skin glue, made up of ceramides and other lipids, in a basketweave pattern. This is actually a good death, as it were, because these cells protect your skin, keeping the elements out and necessary moisture in. But because these cells are dead, they eventually need to be sloughed off.

When you're young, the skin cells renew themselves every two to three weeks. As we age, however, this skin cell renewal and sloughing process slows down . . . and down. (Which is why we need to add exfoliants to our skin-care regimens. This will be discussed in chapter 10.)

Bottom line: Skin needs the gentlest, not the strongest, cleansing that still gets the job done.

UNDERSTANDING SOAPS AND CLEANSERS

When it comes to cleansing our skin there are so many choices it's hard to know what to choose. It helps to know the basics about what cleansers actually are.

Soaps are extracted from plant and animal material, and the result is a complex mixture of chemicals called triglycerides. Variations in the mixture explain why every soap may feel and look different. Add to this colorants and fragrances, and the result can be irritation rather than clean and clear skin.

Since the precise mix of chemicals is not controlled during extraction, soaps often have too much of the few components that are very strong, and this can strip skin of natural oils and leave it dry. And anyone who lives in an area with hard water, which is naturally loaded with a lot of dissolved minerals, knows that soap reacts to the mineral content by forming an annoying film called soap scum.

Soap-free soaps and soap-free cleansers are made with **detergents.** Detergents are made from petrochemicals and come in many shapes,

sizes, and with many different properties. Ironically, detergents synthesized from petrochemicals are usually much more pure than soaps. And
as soap-free soaps are made by mixing together precise combinations of
detergents, they are usually just as effective as soaps when it comes to
washing, but much gentler on dry skin.

Bottom line: While soap manufacturers claim that their soaps are
natural and "pure," bear in mind that soap-free soaps are just as pure
and often easier on your skin.

HOW TO USE CLEANSERS

It is possible to wash your skin too much, especially if you are using
harsh soaps or strong detergents. The only good that comes of this is for
companies that make moisturizers, as you'll need them by the bucket!

Many of us feel inclined to scrub our faces more than necessary because we erroneously believe that pimples result from dirty skin. This is
simply not true, but it has inspired a host of overly zealous cleansers and
created the impression for many that their skin is not truly clean unless
it feels taut and tight and stripped of all oils. Another problem is that for
some people the gentle cleanser that works in the morning is not strong
enough to remove the makeup and grime that's accumulated during the
day. So they opt for a slightly stronger detergent, with the downside that
these stronger detergents take off more than makeup and they often
leave the skin dry. So what can you do?

One recent product trend is the nighttime cleansing cloth, such as
the Dove Facial Cleansing Cloths or the Neutrogena Make-up Remover
Cleansing Towelettes, to remove makeup without soaking the skin in
detergents that strip it of precious oils. Some are premoistened and others must be wetted with warm water. The cloth texture also helps to
gently loosen dirt and all debris. Face scrubs with scrubbing grains are
unnecessarily harsh. If it's exfoliation you want, try the alpha-hydroxy
acid products in chapter 10.

Here are some other suggestions for using cleansers for maximum
skin benefits:

■ Limit the amount of cleansing to no more than twice a day, especially if one of those sessions is needed to remove makeup.

■ Washing your face in the shower or bath with soap counts as cleansing.

■ In the morning, use a gentle cleanser or consider using nothing more than lukewarm water if your skin is dry. Nighttime cleansing to remove makeup may be all that you'll need.

■ Remember, the cleanser is going to be washed away immediately. You don't need one that's loaded with fancy ingredients as you're only paying to wash them down the drain!

■ Keep it simple and basic. Most of the recommended cleansers on the following lists are available in drugstores or beauty stores and are not expensive. You don't need to spend a lot of money on a daytime cleanser unless you really want to.

■ Nighttime cleansers with added ingredients tend to feel more luxurious on the skin. Be aware that although these are good products, once again most of what you're paying for is going to be washed right off.

It may take a little homework and some simple testing to find the best cleanser for you, especially if your skin is oily during part of the month and dry during other weeks. Here's how to find what works for you:

■ Start with the most water-soluble, or rinse-off, cleanser. This property will clearly be stated on the cleanser's label. Benzenesulfonates and stearates are very water soluble and gentle; sodium lauryl sulfate is less water soluble and a strong detergent, and so should be used cautiously.

■ If you don't think the mildest cleanser is working for your skin, you can try a slightly stronger one next. Tip-offs are that you have to rub too hard to remove makeup or you find yourself lathering up a second time.

■ If your skin becomes irritated, uncomfortably tight, or too dry after cleansing, the cleanser you're using is too harsh, you're using too much, or you're washing too frequently. Also, a cleanser shouldn't sting your eyes. Switch back to a milder cleanser.

▓ More cleanser doesn't mean more cleansing. It means drier skin. Use the smallest amount necessary to do the job.

▓ A lather isn't needed for cleansing, so don't choose a soap or cleanser based on the amount of lather you can work up and put on your face.

▓ A stronger detergent soap can be used for the rest of your body. There are more oil glands, and body skin is not as prone to dryness.

▓ Avoid using deodorant soap on your face, as it can be especially drying. The deodorant ingredient is designed to be left on the skin and dry it up to stop the growth of bacteria. Deodorant soaps, such as Irish Spring or Tom's of Maine, are clearly labeled "deodorant."

RECOMMENDED DAYTIME CLEANSERS (MILD)

Remember: ❀ means luxury products and • means drugstore products.

Bar Cleansers
- Basis Sensitive Skin Bar
- Dove Sensitive Skin Beauty Bar
- Purpose Gentle Cleansing Bar

Liquid Cleansers
- Bioré Foaming Liquid Cleanser
- Cetaphil Gentle Daily Cleanser
- Dove Sensitive Skin Foaming Facial Cleanser
- ❀ Estée Lauder Perfectly Clean Foaming Cleanser
- ❀ Garden Botanika Skin Renewing Gentle Foaming Cleanser
- Olay Foaming Face Wash
- ❀ Shiseido Pureness Cleansing Gel

RECOMMENDED NIGHTTIME CLEANSERS (SIMPLE CLEANSING)

Liquid Cleansers

- Aveeno Clear Complexion Foaming Cleanser
- ✿ Clarins Cleansing Milk
- ✿ Clinique Wash-Away Gel Cleanser
- ✿ Dr. Hauschka Cleansing Milk
- Eau Thermale Avène Emollient Cleansing Gel with Cold Cream
- ✿ Givenchy Clean It Tender Creamy Cleansing Foam
- Neutrogena Deep Clean Facial Cleanser
- ✿ Peter Thomas Roth Chamomile Cleansing Lotion
- ✿ T. Leclerc Gentle Cleansing Milk

Cleansing Cloths

- Dove Facial Cleansing Cloths
- Neutrogena Make-up Remover Cleansing Towelettes
- Olay Daily Facials Cleansing Cloths (witch hazel may be irritating for some)

YOUR CHOICE: NIGHTTIME CLEANSERS WITH ADDED INGREDIENTS

I don't really recommend cleansers with additives, but many have a very nice feel despite the wasteful ingredients. If you don't mind spending extra, consider these:

CLEANSER	ADDED INGREDIENTS
✿ DERMAdoctor Wrinkle Revenge Antioxidant Enhanced Glycolic Acid Facial Cleanser	Antioxidants, glycolic acid (three strengths)
✿ Exuviance Purifying Cleansing Gel	AHAs
✿ Joey New York Calm	Vitamin B, vitamin E, aloe vera

and Correct Gentle
Soothing Cleanser
- Mary Kay TimeWise   Vitamin A, vitamin E
  3-in-1 Cleanser
- M.D. Forté Facial   15 percent glycolic acid
  Lotion I
- Murad AHA/BHA   Glycolic and salicylic acid, sodium
  Exfoliating Cleanser   PCA (pyrrolidone carboxylic acid, a
                            natural humectant)

Bottom line: Pick the gentlest cleanser that does the job and don't bother with those with many extra ingredients, unless you are willing to pay for the feel.

ANTIMICROBIAL CLEANSERS

All germs are the enemy, right?

Many types of microbes can and do cause skin infections. But you may be surprised to find out that germs live all over our skin all the time. In fact, there are some good varieties of germs that help keep our skin healthy by forcing out dangerous germs. For example, the relatively weak *Staphylococcus epidermidis* grows on the skin in large numbers, keeping down the numbers of the much more infectious *Staphylococcus aureus*.

The war on germs is certainly a convenient marketing hook, one that's been incredibly successful. Which is why one of the newer salvos in the antimicrobial wars is the category of cleansers and soaps with antimicrobial agents added to the mix.

Antimicrobial cleansers were pioneered in hospitals in the early twentieth century as hand cleansers for busy surgeons, physicians, and nurses. Their original purpose was to stop patient infections that were spread from bacterial contaminants on the hands of caregivers. Study after study has shown that these antimicrobial cleansers are effective in reducing the bacterial load on the hands of hospital workers and in reducing infections among patients. This makes perfect sense in a hospital environment.

. Today, this idea has run amok, and antimicrobials have been added to consumer cleansers and soaps with the idea of protecting the hand washer from bacteria and the kind of viruses that cause colds and the flu. In fact, manufacturers introduced more than 570 new antibacterial products into the consumer market in 2004 and 2005 alone!

And they know who's going to use these cleansers. Some of the heaviest users are mothers with young children, who can be seen spritzing away with their antibacterial hand sanitizer on baby's toys and mom's cell phone. The common ingredient in antimicrobial cleansers is triclosan, a broad-spectrum antibacterial/antimicrobial agent, which has been proven to be a highly effective germ killer. Triclosan also appears in a wide variety of household products, including laundry detergents, deodorants, toothpaste, and mouthwashes. Among the most popular antibacterial cleansers are Colgate-Palmolive Softsoap, Dial Liquid Gold Antimicrobial Soap, and Procter & Gamble's Safeguard.

The problem is that there is very little proof that antimicrobial agents do any good for the average consumer. Procter & Gamble admitted in an August 19, 2003, letter to the U.S. Food and Drug Administration that "the benefits that result from washing with antibacterial soaps cannot be easily measured under consumer use conditions."

In fact, the Columbia University School of Nursing conducted a one-year test in 238 Manhattan households in which they compared a plain hand-washing soap with one containing triclosan. The researchers taught the participants the proper way to wash their hands and monitored their compliance during the study. They found, not surprisingly, that by the end of the study the amount of bacteria found on the hands of the subjects was significantly reduced compared to the levels recorded at the start of the study. That would be expected, because people tend to wash their hands more thoroughly when they are being monitored.

The unexpected result was that it didn't make any difference whether the soap was a plain one or one of the antimicrobial concoctions; each reduced bacterial contamination to an equally low level. The most important factors in cleansing are the time taken and the thoroughness of the cleansing, including under the fingernails. The study concluded, "The risk-benefit ratio argues in favor of targeted rather than ubiquitous, general household use of anti-microbial soap." By "targeted," they meant to restrict the use of antimicrobial soaps to caregivers for those people who are really sick. These antimicrobial soaps don't really protect the hand washer, just the patient.

Some scientists worry that the shotgun approach of these antimicrobial soaps and sprays not only does no particular good, but encourages growth of drug-resistant bacteria that could eventually no longer be killed by triclosan. This would be a serious setback for everyone. Luckily, a one-year study did not find an increase in drug-resistant bacteria among those using antimicrobial soaps. The FDA remains concerned, however, and has convened a committee of experts to monitor the problem.

Still, because so few consumers truly understand the science of dealing with germs, skin-care companies will continue to create products that capitalize on misperceptions and fears. One such product, Probiotic Anti-Stress Lotion from D'Arcy Laboratories, for example, has claimed that it contains the DNA of living beneficial bacteria that destroy toxic bacteria, as well as containing its own beneficial bacteria to replenish the population on skin. This is simply impossible, since DNA cannot kill living bacteria. In fact, bacteria and viruses can instead take over loose DNA and absorb it into one of their own genes. More to the point, the notion of a product packed with living bacteria is quite alarming, since bacterial growth in a cosmetic is a serious health risk.

Bottom line: There is no reason to use any antimicrobial cleansers, unless you are caring for a seriously ill person who is at risk for infection. They should not be used on your face at any time as they are strong and extremely drying. Instead, you are better off sticking to plain cleansing bars for all routine hand washing—and doing a more thorough job of it.

THE TRUTH ABOUT TONERS

For decades, consumers have been told that an essential part of any comprehensive skin-care regimen is a toner, a product that follows the use of a cleanser. Toners were originally designed to remove soap scum, shrink pores, and tighten skin in preparation for makeup. Now there are actually two kinds of toners: those used to finish the cleansing process and those used as moisturizers.

Toners used to finish the cleansing process were called "astringents" and were created to clear off the debris and soap scum left on the face by the soaps and rich cleansing milks popular through the 1970s and 1980s. The idea was to finish the job with a tonic that would close pores and leave a clean slate for makeup. Astringents did their job by producing a slight irritation and swelling of the skin, which in turn did close the tops of the pores.

The problem with these toners is that they're composed primarily of alcohol, acetone, and/or witch hazel, with camphor, menthol, boric acid, rosewater, and alum often added. All these ingredients are incredibly drying. So while many consumers grew to love the temporary smooth and cool feeling they got when they applied a toner—a feeling caused by the rapidly evaporating alcohol and menthol—they had no idea that their pores would not remain closed for long and that they were in essence leaving their skin parched and vulnerable.

Moisturizing toners don't contain the traditional harsh ingredients, such as alcohol or acetone, found in astringent toners but instead contain mostly water and other ingredients that can smooth skin. For example, the Flower Essence Toner from Kiss My Face is made from water, glycerin, and various plant oils. Nivea Visage Moisturizing Toner and L'Oréal Plenitude HydraFresh Toner both have no alcohol and they contain provitamin B_5 to prepare the skin for a moisturizer. This evolution of the toner category is completed by Eucerin Clear Skin Formula Deep Action Toner, which contains lactic acid as its primary active ingredient in an anti-acne skin-care regimen—and actually claims to keep pores *open*. This is the complete opposite of the original astringents, designed to *close* pores!

Today, with cleansing bars favored over soaps, there is even less need for toners, as most people don't need to get rid of soap scum. And if you're looking for extra moisture, simply use a moisturizer instead. A toner is often an unnecessary step and an additional cost.

Bottom line: Whatever toners are called, and whatever their intended use, chances are very slim—unless you are using natural soaps

Cleansers and Toner Ingredients to Avoid

One of the most common tricks of the cosmetic trade is to add a slightly irritating component to a cleanser and then tell the consumer who feels a "tingle" that this is proof that the product is working! The ingredients on this list cause that tingle. They're here because they dry the skin or create an unnecessary irritation. Above all, they do not help the product to work.

Acetone

Alcohol

Alum

Boric acid

Camphor

Eucalyptus

Fragrance

Menthol

Peppermint

Rosewater

Witch hazel

and have hard water—that you need one. In fact, nearly all of them have lost their original purpose. Unless your dermatologist specifically recommends a toner, what you need instead is an effective moisturizer.

■　■　■

Moisturizers

Moisturizers are the weapons in the battlefield of the New Skin-Care Revolution.

Sure, moisturizers have been used for thousands of years, but these traditional products are distant cousins to some of the remarkable new products being launched in the twenty-first century. Formulas can now be modernized so that the basic ingredients remain the same but the effects last much longer. Even better, multitasking moisturizers can now deliver the benefits once found only on a groaning shelf of many different products. The very best moisturizers not only deliver moisture to parched skin, but treat wrinkles, add vitality, and give you a real glow.

THE EARLY GENERATIONS OF MOISTURIZERS

Glamour is not new. Jars of salves have been unearthed in graves from the first Egyptian dynasty, and in ancient Greece, aromatic oils were used before athletic matches, rubbed onto the body after bathing, and used to anoint the heads of nobles. In Roman times Queen Cleopatra had milk poured into her bath as an early exfoliation treatment.

For the next seventeen hundred years, mothers handed down complex recipes for homemade moisturizers to their daughters and apothecaries compounded products at the local pharmacy. In 1872, Robert Chesebrough patented a solution extracted from the muck found on the drilling rigs in oil fields. He promptly dubbed it petroleum jelly, or

Vaseline, and the Chesebrough Manufacturing Company went on to make its fortune selling what had once been unwanted oily gunk and was now the balm that soothed many an irritated baby bottom.

In 1914, the T.T. Pond Company of Utica, New York, introduced a Vanishing Cream to even out skin tone. It was soon joined by Pond's Cold Cream, and they became the cosmetic world's first smash success. Soon, entrepreneurs and impresarios were marketing thick emulsions and soothing, smooth creams to beauty-conscious women. This was the beginning of the moisturizer market. Consumer expectations were raised by elegantly manufactured moisturizers packaged with veiled promises of a perfect complexion and eternal youth.

But at the end of the day the products just didn't deliver. They couldn't do much more than help keep skin moist, which is why they're referred to as humectants, and they ended up with a dubious reputation as being nothing but hope in a jar.

By the 1990s, moisturizers had become eclipsed by endless cartons of stand-alone specialty products with alluring names and supposedly miraculous hero ingredients. Yet instead of the daily skin-care regimen becoming easier, more and more products were added to the mix. Some companies told their customers to work their way through five-, seven-, even ten-step morning rituals! Take Avon's Anew Clinical Line and Wrinkle Corrector: it evolved into the Lift and Tuck, Night Transforming Lift Cream, Day Transforming Lift Cream, Deep Crease Concentrate, Line Eliminator Neo-Retinol Line Plumper, Retroactive+ Skin Optimizer, Ultimate Transforming Lift Eye Cream, Retroactive+ Repair Eye Serum, Repair Body Lotion, and All-in-One Max SPF 15 UVA/UVB Cream!

For busy women on the go, spending all that time in the bathroom applying layers of products was not usually a feasible solution to their skin-care needs. And at the same time, moisturizers in the 1990s began to be labeled with many new descriptive phrases such as "treatment," "complex," "formula," or "hydrating fluid." With so many old-style products, how could a consumer know what really worked?

HOW BASIC MOISTURIZERS WORK

The earliest known moisturizers had simple ingredients and a simple function. They worked by smothering the skin in a thick layer of salve that shut water inside. As a result, the skin plumped up with retained liquid. These simple yet effective moisturizers are still around, in the form of glycerin, mineral oil, and petrolatum.

The problem with simple humectants is that they lack staying power, so skin quickly returns to dryness once they're absorbed. Vaseline petroleum jelly, on the other hand, is widely used in the medical profession to treat wounds and keep them sterile because it stays on and doesn't evaporate until it's wiped off. But it's an impractical ingredient for skin care, as it's greasy to the touch. Plus it stains clothing. (As a lip balm, though, it works well.)

Enter the more evolved generation of moisturizers. Many were packed with plant extracts or other simple compounds like urea that absorb and retain water, but they were still little more than a more user-friendly form of petrolatum. (The extracts may come from exotic or healthy-sounding plants like jojoba, coconut, or safflower, but by the time they are ground down and boiled in water, the pulp that remains is largely cellulose fibers and sugars, and they are all basically the same. Nothing remains of their romantic origins.) Once the moisturizer is applied to the skin, it evaporates quickly, leaving behind a film of these humectants hugging the last remaining drops of moisture. So no matter what ingredients were listed on the moisturizer's jar, their sole function once they landed on the skin was to retain moisture.

Today moisturizers come in many forms:

Creams—white and thick, these are oil-in-water emulsions made with mineral oil or lanolin.

Lotions—translucent and light, they have a high water content and a specialty ingredient, like a silicone, hydrogel, or PEG (polyethylene glycol) to allow them to spread evenly with a smooth feel called "slip."

Gels—clear and thick, they are made with less water than lotions and are composed of long chains of electrically charged chemicals called polymers. Hyaluronic acid, one of the principal moisture-holding natural components of skin, is often used to form a gel that puffs up with water and maintains a jellylike consistency.

Serums—clear, translucent or creamy, but very thin and sometimes runny, serums are formed from water and oil incompletely mixed, or from cyclic silicones. They mix well with skin oils, allowing for easy application of makeup.

Given the assaults that our skin undergoes during the day—weather, pollution, dry indoor environments, dirt, rubbing and poking—all women past the age of about thirty should use some kind of moisturizer, in the morning and at night. Even those with oily skin often need moisturizers, because a healthy skin barrier has a balance of both water and oil. (In skin, the cell glue is made by oil and water forming alternating layers. Too much or too little oil disrupts the glue and breaks the skin barrier.) Only those with severe acne and excessively oily skin should skip moisturizers, and if your skin is very troubled, it is best treated with the guidance of a board-certified dermatologist.

There are lots of good, older-generation moisturizers—that do what they're supposed to do, namely hydrate the skin—available in stores and online. The tried and true can be just as effective and a lot cheaper than many of the new, hugely hyped products, and many of them are multitasking, adding specific ingredients to streamline your daily regimen. Incorporating a sunscreen is also a great way to protect skin from the sun while keeping it hydrated.

RECOMMENDED BASIC MOISTURIZERS

Here are moisturizers that, despite some of their jazzed-up names and lofty promises, should be counted on basically to deliver hydration to the skin.

Facial Use — With Added Sunscreen

- Amway Artistry Time Defiance Day Protect Crème SPF 15
- Dove Deep Moisture Facial Lotion for Dry Skin with SPF 15
- ☀ Estée Lauder DayWear Plus SPF 30
- L'Oréal Advanced RevitaLift Cream or Lotion SPF 15
- L'Oréal Dermo-Expertise Futur*e Moisturizer+ a Daily Dose of Pure Vitamin E SPF 15
- Mary Kay TimeWise Age-Fighting Moisturizer Sunscreen SPF 15
- Neutrogena Healthy Skin Face Lotion SPF 15

- Olay Complete All Day Moisture Lotion SPF 15
- Olay Total Effects 7X Visible Anti-Aging Vitamin Complex with UV Protection (vitamins B_3, B_5, C, and E and sunscreens)
- Pond's Mend & Defend Intensive Protection SPF 15

Facial Use — Without Sunscreen

- Clean & Clear Oil-Free Dual Action Moisturizer (for oily skin and acne, with salicylic acid)
- ☼ Clinique Dramatically Different Moisturizing Lotion
- ☼ H_2O Plus Face Oasis Hydrating Treatment (with vitamins A, C, E, and provitamin B)
- Neutrogena Advanced Solutions Skin Transforming Complex Nightly Renewal Cream (with retinol, for cell renewal; an AHA for exfoliation; and DMAE, a neuropeptide alleged to assist in the production of neurotransmitters to help tone the skin)

Body Use

- Curél Ultra Healing Intensive Moisture Lotion (with glycerin and petrolatum)
- Eucerin Aquaphor (with glycerin)
- Eucerin Calming Cream (with oatmeal and glycerin)
- Jergens Age Defying Multi-Vitamin Moisturizer (with glycerin, cetearyl alcohol, and petrolatum)
- Lubriderm Daily Moisture (with mineral oil, petrolatum, and lanolin; lanolin can be irritating)
- Lubriderm Sensitive Moisture (with butylene glycol, mineral oil, petrolatum, glycerin)
- Mary Kay Time Wise Cellu-Shape Daytime Body Moisturizer
- Neutrogena Norwegian Formula Body Moisturizer (with glycerin)
- ☼ Origins A Perfect World Highly Hydrating Body Lotion (with shea butter)
- Vaseline Intensive Care Firming & Radiance Age-Defying

Lotion (with glycerin, dimethicone, potassium lactate, stearic acid, and mineral oil)

- Vaseline Intensive Care Healthy Body Complexion Nourishing Body Lotion (with glycerin, dimethicone, potassium lactate, stearic acid, and mineral oil)

THE POWER MOISTURIZERS — BUILDING A BETTER BARRIER FROM THE INSIDE OUT

Despite the many good, basic options on the market, you no longer have to make do with a simple moisturizer. Instead, you can up the ante by switching to a power moisturizer created by the technology of the New Skin-Care Revolution—which has proven that moisturizers can and should make a visible difference in your skin. If you begin to use some of these moisturizers you will see results within a few weeks of diligent application.

A power moisturizer is able to use its active ingredients to reprogram the skin to do the following:

1. **Fortify** the topmost skin layers of the stratum corneum by boosting ceramide levels

2. **Calm** inflammation of the middle layers with an effective anti-inflammatory while simultaneously stoking up skin cells with more energy to recover quickly from damage

3. **Increase microcirculation** and **rebuild collagen** in the lower layers

Let's take a look at the best ingredients in the newest generation of moisturizers and how they work. The ones I recommend are purified from botanical extracts, so they have added potency, greater consistency, and are less likely to cause breakouts and irritation.

REJUVENATING THE TOPMOST LAYERS

The older generation of moisturizers could do little more than temporarily boost your skin's water content. A better, long-term solution is to encourage your skin to produce more lipids, or natural oils, on its own as if it were younger skin. By shoring up the topmost layer (the stratum corneum), your skin will look fresher, less wrinkled, and more vibrant. It will literally be rejuvenated!

Ursolic Acid

A few special herbs, spices, and fragrances have within them an uncanny capacity to literally reprogram your DNA and turn back the clock, in some studies by up to thirty years. One ingredient in particular to look for is ursolic acid, from the same chemical family as boswellic acid (the pentacyclic triterpenes, in case you're interested!), found in the boswellia tree. Ursolic acid gives frankincense its soothing properties for arthritis, and its relative, glycyrrhizin, is what gives licorice root its reputation for fighting stomach upset.

Ursolic acid is also found in the waxy covering of the leaves of the rosemary, sage, and heather plants, as well as in the waxy skin of apples, and is what gives rosemary its well-known status as an anti-inflammatory and calming agent. More than three hundred different skin-care products containing extract of rosemary are for sale online. But as I discussed in chapter 3, knowing that rosemary calms inflammation isn't the same as having a ursolic acid derived from rosemary that is potent and purified enough in your product to work on your skin. Look for products with rosemary or sage extract that explicitly mention ursolic acid.

When our lab was testing different rosemary extracts, we discovered something remarkable: ursolic acid redirected the cells to make more lipids! Not just any lipid but, specifically, ceramides and their related lipids—crucial to maintaining the velvety texture of young, plumped-up skin. Ursolic acid is notoriously finicky to work with, so we put it in liposomes, a microscopic lipid sphere, hoping for better delivery into the skin. Well, we soon started testing our version of a ursolic acid cream in a controlled clinical study (and there was no shortage of volunteers!). At the end we were astonished to find that in the skin treated with the ursolic acid liposome lotion, the amount of ceramides and other skin lipids had increased 30 percent (the same 30 percent it decreases from age thirty to age sixty). It was as if this lotion could build skin's outer layer back up—literally rejuvenating the barrier and restoring skin suppleness.

RECOMMENDED MOISTURIZERS WITH URSOLIC ACID

- Avon Anew Alternative Intensive Age Treatment SPF 25 Day
- Charmzone Wrinklear Cream
- Natura Bissé Diamond Body Cream
- Pola Day+Day Vitax Wrinkle Shot
- Remergent Barrier Repair Formula
- Ren Frankincense and *Boswellia Serrata* Revitalising Repair Cream
- Sisley Global Anti-Age Cream

The B Vitamins: Niacinamide and Panthenol

The use of B vitamins, such as niacinamide (a derivative of vitamin B_3) and panthenol (pro-vitamin B_5), in moisturizers is gaining scientific support.

The B vitamins are essential in the diet to avoid disease, but in the skin they don't act like vitamins. Rather, they physically reorder the upper layers of the stratum corneum. In particular, niacinamide has many exfoliating properties similar to the alpha-hydroxy acids, while panthenol is a humectant, keeping moisture locked into the skin. A recent, well-designed study of fifty women who used a high concentration of 5 percent niacinamide for twelve weeks found a reduction in fine lines and wrinkles. They also observed an improvement in skin tone, with fewer hyperpigmentation spots as well as reduced blotchiness and sallowness.

RECOMMENDED MOISTURIZERS WITH B VITAMINS

- Aveeno Active Naturals Positively Radiant Anti-Wrinkle Cream
- H_2O Plus Face Oasis Hydrating Treatment
- Lumene Vitamin+ Vita-Nectar Vitalizing Day Cream SPF 15

- Olay Regenerist Continuous Night Recovery Moisturizing Treatment
- Olay Total Effects 7X Visible Anti-Aging Vitamin Complex

CALMING INFLAMMATION AND IRRITATION

Inflammation is now recognized in all fields of medicine as an underlying cause of many of the chronic conditions of aging, from arthritis to Alzheimer's disease to heart attacks.

In short spurts, inflammation is an essential response by the body to keep out infection. It begins when there's a wound where cells have been killed in a local area and bacteria and viruses can invade the bloodstream. The surrounding cells immediately recognize this as a danger signal, triggering a tidal wave of responses by immune cells.

These immune cells send out chemical signals that attract white blood cells like sharks to bait, which then disgorge a toxic mixture of hydrogen peroxide and other killer chemicals to destroy the invaders. Some of these chemicals also cause the blood vessels to enlarge in order to bring in more white blood cells, which in turn raises the temperature of the wound site and also kills more invaders.

The result? Some collateral damage in the form of inflammation. This is unavoidable, as the hydrogen peroxide and toxins released by the white blood cells destroy normal tissue along with the bacteria. Soon, however, order is restored as your body miraculously cleans up the mess. The reaction subsides and the wound heals.

When it comes to the skin's aging process, inflammation is an underappreciated trigger, caused over the years by repeated cycles of damage and recovery. The inflammatory response that comes about as a result of sun exposure causes the most frequent and the most serious damage to skin. In fact, the damage done by solar radiation in the form of UVA and UVB rays creates microscars, the microscopic remnants of even the most mild of sunburns. (I'll discuss more about what sun does to skin in chapter 6.) Microscars are the first step toward a permanent wrinkle. Because of the damage caused by inflammation, anti-inflammatories are a central part of the best new products that will be coming to the forefront in the New Skin-Care Revolution.

Botanical Anti-Inflammatories

Unfortunately, cosmetics companies to date have not succeeded in developing anti-inflammatory botanicals that truly have a healing effect on irritated skin. The most widely used plant derivative is bisabolol, the active ingredient in chamomile. The leaves of the chamomile plant, a member of the daisy family, have a longstanding reputation as having soothing, anti-inflammatory properties, from chamomile teabags that soothe tired eyes to a light green chamomile plaster smothering the itchy lesions from chicken pox.

But despite chamomile's popularity, and the assertion by herbologists that hundreds of studies have proven the plant's benefits, a careful search of the medical literature reveals no controlled clinical studies that confirm either chamomile or bisabolol as having a potent anti-inflammatory effect when applied to human skin at concentrations available in products from the cosmetic counter or the health food store. The same is also true for aloe and licorice, also "well known" for their soothing properties.

I was determined to find a different plant with anti-inflammatory properties, and our laboratory decided to research the Chinese elixir Wu Zhu Yu (pronounced *woo-shoo-yoo*), used for centuries as a calming tea for upset stomachs as well as the treatment of pain. It's made from the unripe fruit of the *Evodia rutaecarpa* plant grown only in China's southern region. Just before the two annual harvests in August and November, some green berries are gathered, dried in the sun to a dark greenish-brown, then soaked in hot water and licorice juices to make a pungent, bitter tea.

For nearly two years we tried to make a consistent and appealing extract from the evodia plant that could be used in moisturizers, but variation in the quality of the unripe berries made this impossible. Finally, we analyzed the calming ingredients in the extract and prepared a biomimetic, or a lab-created mixture of compounds at the same concentration as found in the original Wu Zhu Yu extract, and with the same anti-irritating qualities. This evodia extract proved more potent than chamomile in clinical studies and became one of the star ingredients in our Remergent Barrier Repair Formula.

There remains a serious need for other calming agents in moisturizers, especially those that tone down inflammation. There are many botanical extracts, such as kukui nut, karite (also known as shea butter), macadamia nut, and avocado oil, which have been studied for their anti-inflammatory properties, with promising results. Be aware that what you can buy over the counter may indeed be based on one of these botanical extracts but may contain such low concentrations that they will have little or no effect on your skin.

Bottom line: Products with proven anti-inflammatory properties are few and far between. The reputation of an ingredient is no guarantee that the right amount is in a product. New products that work are just now coming to market and are listed here.

RECOMMENDED CALMING MOISTURIZERS

- Eucerin Redness Relief Soothing Night Creme (with lichocalcone from licorice root)
- Laboratoire Remède Post Peel Skin Calming Balm (with bisabolol)
- Lindi Soothing Balm (formulated for cancer patients, with avocado oil)
- Oils of Aloha Kukui Essential AfterSun Lotion (with kukui oil and macadamia nut oil)
- Remergent Barrier Repair Formula (with ursolic acid and evodia extract)

Steroids

Pharmaceutical companies have rolled out billion-dollar blockbuster drugs to control inflammation, such as statins and NSAIDs (non-steroidal anti-inflammatory drugs). Skin-care companies, however, have been slow to pick up on this new wave of technology. Instead, they've relied heavily on an outdated repertoire of anti-inflammatory drugs called steroids, left over from the last generation of drugs. These have been divided into four classes:

- Mild steroids, such 0.5% or 1% hydrocortisone (available over the counter)
- Low potency, such as 0.05% desonide

- Mid potency, such as 0.1% betamethasone
- Potent, such as 0.05% clobetasol (this drug is six hundred times as potent as hydrocortisone)

Topical steroids should only be used over a limited period of time, typically a few weeks. Prolonged use can cause side effects such as skin thinning, stretch marks, and easy bruising.

Bottom line: Because using steroids can be dangerous, they are never included in moisturizers. Avoid using them on your face unless directed to do so by your dermatologist.

INCREASING SKIN VITALITY

One of the most common complaints about skin, after dryness, is a loss of vitality—that skin looks and feels tired, as if mental and physical weariness were literally on display for the world to see. Loss of vitality and that blah look may, in fact, be a sign not only that the skin is over-worked—having used up all its reserves of energy—but that it could be hungry, too. Yes, hungry!

Skin is a living organ, after all, and there's a beehive of activity going on in the dermis and epidermis. But skin lacks one critical element that every other organ of the body has—its own complete blood supply. Blood vessels normally do not reach the surface of the skin, which is why a superficial cut or scrape draws no blood. Instead, blood vessels are embedded in the dermis, the lower layer of skin.

It's important to understand just how crucial this distinction is. Instead of the vital oxygen and nutrients being received in the skin by blood transport, they're diffused upward from those buried blood vessels. This is not a terribly efficient process, and it only worsens with age. Measurements of blood flow in the skin surface, either in the arms or the abdomen, show a 30 percent decline from the age of thirty to the age of sixty. Anyone of a certain age who's chronically cold isn't making it up. Less blood flow means less nutrition is available to the skin. And who wants to live with tired and hungry skin if you don't have to?

The good news is that skin starved for oxygen and nutrients can actually be "fed." Not with quackery, but with products loaded with nutrients created in the New Skin-Care Revolution. (See chapter 9 for more about antioxidants.) Stress relief—exercise, recreation, meditation, yoga, and massage—will also improve your skin's appearance, not only because you feel and look more relaxed, but because the improved circulation is great for getting food to your skin.

Because few consumers really understand how to improve circulation to the skin to rejuvenate it, all kinds of bogus solutions, such as yohimbine and ground rhino horn, have been touted over the years. One dubious solution promoted in the 1990s was to add magnetic microparticles to cosmetics. The theory was that since hemoglobin (the chemical in blood that carries oxygen) contains iron, applying a magnetic field to the skin should attract hemoglobin and nourish the skin. The idea is tempting, but if it were true, putting a magnet on the skin would make it turn red, which it does not. In fact, in a clinical study, twelve people had a disk placed on their forearms. One disk was charged with a strong magnetic field, and the other was a placebo. No difference was found in the blood flow at the sites of the two instruments. Similar studies have not found any benefit of magnets for pain, either. Nevertheless, magnetic masks are still hawked for skin treatments.

Skin-cell performance can be improved by borrowing a technique used for decades by body builders—no, not steroids, but amino acids. One amino acid that's been highly touted is carnitine. It works by helping the skin cells burn food more efficiently and make more energy. But its side effect is that while it "heats up" energy production, it can also produce oxygen free radicals that damage cells. Far better than carnitine is ergothioneine, an extraordinarily powerful antioxidant that's very similar to carnitine in structure. Ergothioneine has carnitine's benefits, while providing antioxidant activity to "cool down" the cells during peak energy production. It's made even more effective when combined with vitamin C, so it's important that the two be formulated together. Skin cells produce their own ergothioneine receptors to capture and retain this amino acid within the cell. I'll discuss ergothioneine in greater detail in chapter 9.

RECOMMENDED ERGOTHIONEINE MOISTURIZERS WITH VITAMIN C

* Cellex-C Advanced-C Neck Firming Cream
* Cellex-C Advanced-C Serum
* Cellex-C Advanced-C Skin Tightening Cream
* Remergent Antioxidant Refoliator
* Remergent Barrier Repair Formula
* Remergent Clarifying Concentrate

RECOMMENDED ERGOTHIONEINE MOISTURIZERS WITHOUT VITAMIN C

* Botage 10B Advanced Facial Anti-Oxidant Formula
* Dior No-Age Essentiel Progress Age-Defense Refining Creme
* Kinerase Hydrating Antioxidant Mist
* Kinerase Lip Treatment
* Neways NightScience
* Neways Rebound
* Neways Retention Plus
* Neways Skin Enhancer

DIMINISHING DARK CIRCLES

Dark circles under the eyes are a perennial problem for many women, one that can be especially troubling, as they cause people to automatically assume you're exhausted or stressed!

For years, skin biologists thought that dark under-eye circles were caused by weak circulation in the area, which has naturally thinner skin than the rest of the face. The only available treatment was vitamin K, in formulations similar to those for treating spider veins and broken capillaries. This vitamin, produced by bacteria in the intestines and then distributed throughout the body, is essential for blood clotting. Without it, there can be excessive bleeding and even hemorrhaging after an injury. There have been several clinical studies demonstrating that when added to some skin creams, vitamin K can help clot the blood and block its

Aromatherapy

Aromatherapy has its origins in the perfume industry, but growing clinical evidence demonstrates a link between what we smell, how we feel, and the way our skin looks. So it makes sense that aromatherapy can have a positive effect on our bodies through the signals sent through the nose to the brain.

Aromatherapy can be used in many different ways, from scents pulsed into the air through sprays, diffusers, heated essential oils, or products applied to the skin. (Pure essential oils should always be diluted prior to application on the skin, as they are extremely potent and can be irritating in their raw state.) Moisturizers with powerful scents are usually recommended for stress relief. Recent research has even suggested that some fragrances, like lavender, can help some people lose weight.

Properties of Popular Essential Oils

Bay laurel	Confidence building
Bergamot	Cheering, fighting depression and fatigue
Frankincense	Calming
Jasmine	Calming
Lavender oil	Calming, promoting weight loss
Rosemary	Energizing
Sandalwood	Calming, confidence building
Ylang-ylang	Calming

flow. But part of the problem with vitamin K is that it's notoriously unstable. As a result, formulas that work in the lab or during clinical studies may not be effective after the product sits for a while in a warehouse or on a store shelf.

The New Skin-Care Revolution, with its emphasis on molecular biology, has turned the thinking about dark under-eye circles on its head. Rather than trying to close off blood flow under the eyes with vitamin K, the new approach is to *stimulate* blood flow. This flushes away the purplish dark color of stagnant veins and reduces the puffiness of slow-moving lymph drainage. The technology is based on the 1998 Nobel

RECOMMENDED AROMATHERAPY PRODUCTS

✿ Dead Sea Salts Relaxing Lavender Aromatherapy Bath Salt
✿ Jason Meditation Masque Aromatherapy
✿ Kaori Revitalizing Ylang Ylang Body Lotion
✿ Lancôme Aroma Tonic spray
✿ Origins Peace of Mind Cease and Destress Diffuser
✿ Origins Peace of Mind Sensory Therapy

ESSENTIAL OILS AND FRAGRANCES TO AVOID

All of these aromatherapy oils carry a high risk of causing irritation or allergic reactions:

Bitter almond oil

Camphor oil

Deertongue oil

Mugwort oil

Pennyroyal oil

Spanish broom oil

Sweet birch oil

Wormseed oil

Wormwood oil

Prize–winning discovery of the small molecule nitric oxide's effects on stimulating blood flow (similar to what nitroglycerin can do during heart attacks, when it temporarily opens closed arteries). Our lab decided to take a close look at two botanical compounds from a chemical family called bicyclic monoterpene diols ("diols" for short) that stimulate production of nitric oxide.

The results of an experiment amazed us. Six volunteers applied our diol cream on one cheek and left the other cheek bare. Then they put on winter coats with no hoods or hats and went into our refrigerated storage room, about 40°F, and shivered for half an hour. When they came out, we immediately measured the temperature of each cheek and found that in every person, the diol-treated cheek was distinctly warmer than the untreated cheek! This is exactly what should happen if the diol cream really did increase microcirculation. It kept the skin warmer in the cold environment.

In our next clinical study, we had twenty-six subjects apply a diol cream twice a day under only their right eye. After four weeks, trained observers who did not know which eye was treated identified the diol-treated side as showing improvement, and overall they measured a statistically significant difference between the treated and untreated eyes. We published both of these studies in a scientific journal specializing in nitric oxide.

Even better, we've since found that nitric oxide can increase collagen production. This is definitely an ingredient that's going to help many people's skin in a big way in the near future.

Bottom line: For many people, dark under-eye circles are caused by slow blood flow, and new products are available that help.

RECOMMENDED VITAMIN K PRODUCTS

- Dermal-K Clarifying Cream
- Dermalogics Eyederma
- Donell Skin Care K-Derm Gel or Cream (formerly known as Super-Skin)
- Jason Vitamin K Crème Plus
- Skin Amnesty Regenerating Eye Cream

RECOMMENDED DIOL PRODUCTS

- Remergent Microcirculation Therapy

THE TRUTH ABOUT CELLULITE

It's time to sit down and talk about cellulite.

Now, you might be wondering why I'd include this is in a chapter on moisturizers. The reason is simple: most of the products created to "treat" cellulite are nothing more than moisturizers with added ingredients.

Far too many of these products overpromise and underdeliver, entreating and enticing the countless millions of women, no matter how thin and toned they are, who suffer from the embarrassing ripples of cellulite. And they're desperate for any product that can make cellulite disappear for good.

Cellulite is formed by fat deposited just under the collagen fibers that support the skin and hold the muscles in place. These fibers are bundled together in a sort of mesh grid. When the fat pushes its way through this grid, it creates ripples and dimples (and a lot of angst). Women will always be more prone to cellulite than men because they tend to have a higher ratio of body fat to muscle, and they accumulate cellulite in places, like the buttocks, hips, and thighs, that are proportionately wider than they are in men.

Cellulite-reduction products are designed to increase circulation, which in turn is supposed to increase fat-cell metabolism. These products rely on a group of compounds called methylxanthines, which includes caffeine. Unfortunately, neither drinking copious cups of coffee nor slathering on caffeine-enriched creams is a cure for cellulite. Worse, no convincing evidence has ever been presented for more than a few millimeters of change in girth with the use of any of these products.

The most common short-term quick fix for cellulite is a product that will dehydrate the skin, stretching it taut over the bumps and thereby minimizing them. However, this is an unhealthy solution that has no lasting effect.

Many other unproven techniques, such as deep-tissue massage and various devices to increase circulation, will continue to crowd the marketplace with claims that they're the real deal at long last. Some tantalizing new evidence is emerging that an FDA-approved device that directs radio waves to cellulite, called VelaSmooth, might help, but as this device is so new, it's too early to tell if it really works. Laser breakup of fat, called laser lipolysis, is now being performed by the Cynosure Smart Lipo laser with encouraging results, but only for small areas. For some women, a diet that reduces fat and fluid retention, combined with exercise, will help.

The only long-term OTC solutions, so far, seem to be those products that strengthen collagen production, which will tighten the mesh of the supporting fibers, reducing the load of fat tissue that bulges through. Moisturizers with strong collagen-building ingredients, like vitamin A, vitamin C, and diols, should help. But you need to give them at least eight weeks to see any change.

RECOMMENDED COLLAGEN BUILDERS

- Cellex-C Advanced-C Serum
- MD Formulations Vit-A-Plus
- Remergent Microcirculation Therapy
- RoC Retinol Correxion Deep Wrinkle Daily Moisturizer
- SkinCeuticals C E Ferulic

DON'T-BELIEVE-THE-HYPE MOISTURIZER INGREDIENTS

Bluster and overpromising are rampant among moisturizer promotions, where fads and "hero" ingredients are touted by doctors using scientific jargon but offering little or no evidence of effectiveness. Here are some overhyped ingredients to watch out for.

CARNITINE

Carnitine is a simple amino acid, one of the building blocks of protein and part of the natural machinery that produces energy for cells. It's used by bodybuilders who want to put on muscle mass quickly. Unfortunately, as it turns up energy production it also increases cellular free radicals, which damage the cell machinery that makes more energy.

Unfortunately, and contrary to the claims made by some dermatologists such as Dr. Adrienne Denese and Dr. Nicholas Perricone, carnitine is not a very effective antioxidant, and it can't stop the out-of-control free radical process. (For more about free radicals, see chapter 9.) There is a much more effective form of carnitine—ergothioneine. This is the ingredient you should be looking for.

CERAMIDES

Ceramides are, as you know by now, the sticky, oily lipid chemicals that bind skin cells together in a kind of mesh on the topmost layer of your skin, the stratum corneum. On a molecular level, ceramide-producing genes shut down over the years, so that your skin produces fewer ceramides and gets visibly dry. Clinical studies support this assertion, showing a steady fall in the strength of the stratum corneum over time—it drops about 30 percent as you age from thirty to sixty.

Ceramides are a common ingredient in many different moisturizers, whether they come in high-priced glass jars or mass-market tubes. Loading ceramides into formulas is a well-meaning solution to the problem—one that, unfortunately, doesn't quite work. For one thing, several aromatic oils, such as jojoba, borage, coconut, or safflower, often contain ceramides that absolutely do lubricate the skin, but in order for them to have any effect, you'd end up looking like a shiny greaseball. More important, simply adding ceramides to a cream doesn't mean they'll penetrate your skin where they're needed. Ceramides are produced *inside* skin cells, which wait for signals to weave them into the skin barrier. When the cells get the signal that's been preprogrammed into your DNA, ceramides are released just as the skin cells migrate upward to a few layers below the surface. Ceramides added onto the skin get absorbed only into the topmost dead layers of the stratum corneum—but they can't get down to the lower levels where they're needed the most. Any relief provided by topical ceramides is fleeting and the results not much better than other moisturizers.

HEAVY METALS: COPPER AND CHELATORS

Copper is a natural metal and is found in small amounts throughout the body. The copper peptide craze, led by the Neutrogena Visibly Firm line of day and night products, is based on claims that more copper will do your skin some good. Interesting research was published some time ago about using copper to treat burns and increase wound healing, but unfortunately since then it's hard to find any evidence from Neutrogena supporting antiwrinkle or moisturizing claims for copper.

On the other hand, according to Dr. Dennis F. Gross, too much of any metal in the skin is bad, and he advocates chelation therapy. Chelators are chemicals that bind tightly to metals and take them out of circulation. Dr. Gross's MDSkincare line offers a Hydra-Pure Intense Moisture Cream that features the "Hydra-Pure Chelating Complex," which Dr. Gross claims removes heavy metal left by water on the skin. Dr. Gross has not made available his findings that his chelating complex improves skin.

One thing is clear—don't use Neutrogena Visibly Firm and Dr. Gross's products at the same time! In the end, neither side has much scientific support, so don't be snowed by these products.

KINETIN

Some esoteric plant-derived ingredients are highly touted as new technology, but in reality they aren't much more than simple moisturizers. One such ingredient is kinetin, whose chemical name is N^6-furfuryladenine. It's the active ingredient in Kinerase, made by Valeant Pharmaceuticals.

Kinetin, a plant hormone belonging to a group called cytokinins, was first isolated in 1955. Bear in mind that plant hormones are not the same as animal or human hormones, but some laboratory experiments with cultured animal cells have shown that cytokinins may stimulate cell division. This has led to the description of kinetin as a "growth factor." Sadly, this is a bit of an exaggeration. Many types of nutrients, such as proteins, sugars, and salts, also stimulate cell growth, but we would hardly give them such an exalted title.

A careful look at the scientific evidence presented by Kinerase shows that kinetin helps skin retain water—which makes it an effective moisturizer, but not much else. No convincing clinical studies have shown that there are any clinical benefits for kinetin in humans beyond moisturization.

NEUROPEPTIDES

"Neuropeptides" are ingredients that have been highly touted, especially by Dr. Nicholas Perricone. Basically, a neuropeptide is a very small protein chain that fits snugly onto a nerve cell and causes it to fire out a burst of neurotransmitters. The explanation for their supposed benefit is that when the neuropeptides are rubbed on skin, they trigger the skin nerves to send out neurotransmitters to the nerves in the muscles in the skin, which then contract and, *voilà*, the skin is firmed.

There are many different types of neuropeptides, and neuroscientists have not yet figured out how each of them works to control nerves. Therefore, it seems unlikely that companies really know which ones (and how much) to put in their products.

Furthermore, it doesn't sound like a good idea to keep skin stretched taut in a perpetual state of stress, since this is when blood flow is constricted, the immune system is suppressed, and skin becomes prone to disease. The tightening explanation doesn't make sense either, because wrinkles disappear in skin *relaxed* by Botox, so you might expect neuropeptides actually to accentuate wrinkles!

There is no evidence that skin-care products either contain any true and effective neuropeptides or get anywhere near real nerves. Don't be taken in by this expensive pseudoscience hype.

MOISTURIZER INGREDIENTS TO AVOID
Some exotic-sounding ingredients that are added to moisturizers actually make things worse. Be careful of too many "natural" extracts, any of which could contain "natural" irritants. For example, irritants like menthol, mint, and peppermint—which may sound appealing—are included to give a tingling feeling so you think the product is working. Methyl nicotinate is a chemical that gives a quick red blush to the skin, making you think that the product is active when it may not be. Both tingling and blushing reactions are caused by aggravating the skin and nothing more.

Known Irritants
Ethanol
Fragrances
Glycerin
Lanolin

Menthol
Methyl nicotinate
Mint
Peppermint
Propylene glycol
Sorbitol

■   ■   ■

Sun Care: It's Never Too Late

Just as the sun warms the earth and brings forth life, it also takes life away—especially from your skin. No one can dispute the unfortunate fact that the ultraviolet (UV) component of sun exposure is the overriding cause of wrinkles, sagging, splotches, blotches, dark spots, flaking, and worn-out skin—what we call photoaging.

Overall, sun protection is by far the most effective anti-aging treatment for people of all ages. If proof is needed of what photoaging has done to your skin, place your forearm next to your inner thigh and notice the difference. The result of what you thought was a "healthy" tan is not bronzed skin but actual damage to the vital DNA in your cells. Damage that accelerates the aging process—yet is almost entirely preventable.

Remember, you can spend thousands of dollars on the most expensive skin-care products or on visits to the dermatologist for injections of fillers, but if you go out in the sun unprotected, you're just throwing away your money and ruining your skin!

Defense against UV rays, until very recently, was completely dependent on sunscreens. When they're used properly—and few consumers know how to do this, but you'll learn how starting in this chapter—sunscreens *will* prevent skin from getting burned after a day at the beach. They will prevent tans from forming. And they will reduce photoaging.

Armed with that knowledge, however, a large part of the medical and scientific profession declared victory over UV radiation and abandoned the sun protection battlefield, leaving mothers to plead in vain with their children to use sunscreens while forgetting to put them on themselves. Despite the widespread availability of sunscreens, the rate of skin cancer continues to grow, and every year more than one-third of Americans report getting a sunburn. Only recently has it become clear that we've hit the wall with sunscreens, and we've realized that they're not the last word in sun protection. A dependence on sunscreens alone to stop photoaging and skin cancer is clearly not working.

Now, by tackling sun protection needs with molecular biology, the New Skin-Care Revolution offers an entirely new approach to managing the effects of sun exposure, including boosting the immune system. By far the most promising treatment is one that optimizes your skin's own natural DNA repair. It has become possible to "clean your genes" and literally reverse decades of UV damage. It is absolutely wrong to believe that once the sun has damaged your skin, nothing more can be done. Sunscreens are the first defense, and new sun protection is in the New Skin-Care Revolution. The ideal time to repair the sun damage and prepare for the future is *now*—whatever your age and whatever state of disrepair your skin may be in. **It is never too late to repair sun damage today and start protecting for tomorrow.**

First, let's take a look at what UV radiation is, how the sun damages skin, and what sunscreens are. Then I'll go into detail about the new products you can use to give your skin the ultimate in sun protection.

UVA AND UVB PRIMER

UVA and UVB are different wavelengths of light, just like green light differs from red light. UVA is about twenty times more abundant than UVB on the earth's surface, but UVB produces a thousand times more damage than UVA.

One way to think about UVA and UVB is to imagine driving a car through a construction site. Nails carelessly dropped are scattered all around. Most of the nails are short (UVA) and inflict only a little damage to the tires, and are unlikely to cause a flat until quite a few are struck. A few of the nails are long, thick, and sharp (UVB), and even a single one can cause a flat. It might be a good idea to pick up the short nails from the road, but without cleaning up the long nails the real dangers remain.

A widely held view, repeated by many dermatologists and in cited articles about the sun, is that UVB damages DNA and causes sunburn, while UVA produces free radicals and causes aging. There's even a catchy slogan: "UVB is for Burning, and UVA is for Aging."

But this misconception has been disproved both in lab experiments and in human testing during the past thirty years. UVB is definitely the more devious villain, as it's more effective than UVA in producing both DNA damage *and* free radicals. That is because UVB slams into skin with far more energy. UVB also causes much worse sunburns and produces much darker tanning than UVA.

Experiments with mice have clearly shown that UVB, on its own, ages the skin and produces deep wrinkling. Even if it was possible to expose skin only to UVB, it would become just as damaged, and maybe more, than if the light only came from UVA. In fact, while both UVA and UVB shut down the skin's immune cells, UVB does so with more thoroughness, which is why carefully controlled doses of artificial UVB have been used since the 1920s for treating serious cases of psoriasis and eczema—diseases involving overactive immune cells that do not respond to topical ointments.

But this does not mean that UVA is by any means safe. A cranked-up blast of UVA that creates a tan will produce the same chemical changes in skin and its DNA that are produced by UVB. Some unscrupulous tanning parlors boast that their UV light machines only produce UVA and therefore are not harmful. This is a dangerous misunderstanding that can cause serious long-term damage to skin—even cancers.

Don't think you're safe from UVA and UVB in your home, office, or cars. Just take a look at the upholstery on a chair near a window to see what the sun can do! Window glass in homes, offices, and cars can screen out some UVA. Car windshield glass blocks about 97 percent of UVA and UVB, but side windows block only one-third to one-half of UVA and UVB.

Bottom line: All forms of UV, including UVA and UVB, produce

DNA damage, cause free radicals to form, cause wrinkling and photoaging, and lead to skin cancer. Protection against UVB is the first priority. Protection against UVA is a second priority, but it must also be part of any effective anti-aging program.

HOW UV RAYS DAMAGE THE SKIN

When you stand in front of a mirror, the face looking back at you is a road map tracing the route your lifelong contest with the sun has taken. This is what you're likely to see:

■ On the surface, skin has thickened. Extra layers of dead skin cells pile up, which reduce clarity and make you look sallow.

■ Pigment cells have cranked out and dispersed their color, trying in vain to deflect the daily UV onslaught. This causes pigmented brown spots (hyperpigmentation) to appear, either as small freckles or as blotchiness. Where all the pigment cells have been killed off by sunlight, white spots appear instead.

■ Deeper inside, injured cells try to heal themselves by squirting digestive enzymes into the supporting layer of collagen and elastin. There, the blood vessels dilate to bring more nutrients to the wounded tissue. Eventually, in some areas, the digested collagen and elastin are spent. They sag and form wrinkles, and the expanded blood vessels squeeze through to the surface so that reddish and bluish veins appear.

But don't give up yet. Molecular biology has made a major advance in our knowledge of sun damage by studying the first few seconds of this conflict—when the sun's rays make their initial strike and hit the skin's DNA.

DNA DAMAGE

DNA, as you know by now, is the basis for how your body works, and every cell is preprogrammed with instructions for its necessary activities. When sunlight strikes the chemicals that make up your DNA, two of its parts can be fused together, like two pages of a book stuck together. (It is important to note here that this reaction does not involve any free radicals—it is direct absorption of the UV light by DNA. This point will be crucial later in chapter 9.) The result is that the coded instructions in the "page" of the DNA manual cannot be read, and control of the cell's activities is blocked. At the same time, the transfer of hereditary information to the next generation of cells is hobbled. It doesn't take many chemical reactions of this type to cripple DNA, and often these stuck-together pages are buried among millions of normal parts of DNA.

We know that cells immediately respond to DNA damage by unleashing a complex of repair enzymes designed to hunt down and patch up the damage. But this is an enormously challenging task for these enzymes, as if searching for a single golden thread in a Persian rug. The process takes time, and time is of the essence. A day after a sunburn, the skin has removed only about half the DNA damage. By the second day, one-quarter of the damage still remains. Eventually, if enough time goes by, a cell with broken DNA is bound to duplicate itself, as cells do, but to do so it has to skip past the damage. This often produces a copying error—which changes the DNA code itself.

Most of the time, these mistakes just kill off the cell, which will be replaced by an undamaged cell. But when that doesn't happen, the wrong change in the code for the wrong gene sends the cell down a path that leads to photoaging and skin cancer. This is why preventing DNA damage is so crucial for anyone who wants to look and feel young and vital (and stay cancer free).

The DNA repair process slows down with age, in everybody. This starts when people hit their twenties, and as years go by, the time needed to rid the cells of damage becomes longer and longer. This means that sun damage to DNA in childhood is almost completely repaired by the time you're a young adult—but the little that remains has decades to fester.

Bottom line: The most serious damage sunlight does to skin is to break down the DNA, and most of this damage does not involve free radicals. We have a natural repair process to fix this, but it's not perfect, and it slows down with age.

STRESS SIGNALS

Scientists have found that even small amounts of UV exposure—the kind you'd get while walking to an appointment or running errands—damages your DNA. Cells with sun-damaged DNA send out stress signals to the surrounding tissue, in the form of tiny molecules called cytokines. There are dozens of different types of cytokines, and they travel near (within the skin) and far (throughout the body) to seek out interested cells and announce the damage by binding to them.

Each target cell responds to the arrival of the stress signal, often by traveling back to the site and releasing toxins designed to sterilize the wounded tissue. Following a large UV dose, these stress signals attract enough responders within twenty-four hours to produce what you recognize as a sunburn.

As I explained in the previous section, the release of the stress cytokines triggers a wound-healing response, highlighted by the release of digestive enzymes, called collagenase and elastase, in the dermis. These enzymes are vital for healing, because they debride your wounds (meaning that they clear away dead tissue to make room for new skin).

The problem is that the minute amounts of collagenase and elastase released deep in the skin after UV exposure also digest bits and pieces of the sturdy collagen and the stretchy elastin that you need for skin suppleness and strength. Your body can only make a little new collagen and elastin to replace what is lost. And with each new exposure, a bit more pigment is released to protect the wounded spot.

The resulting injury is not really noticeable—it's called a "microscar." On its own, a microscar is not a major concern. But over the years, repeated cycles of microscarring turn into very real and very visible damage to the supporting structure of the skin. Say hello to wrinkles, sagging, and age spots.

What's so important to understand is that sunlight doesn't have to reach the lower levels of skin to start the wrinkle process. It only has to reach the upper layers, which then send out the cytokine signals that begin the attack on the lower layers of collagen and elastin. This crucial point is where I firmly disagree with dermatologists who claim that UVA must be the cause of wrinkles because it penetrates to the lower skin layers more easily than does UVB. *Absolutely wrong!* UVB is a much stronger trigger of collagenase and elastase than UVA, because it causes so much more DNA damage (whether it's in the upper or lower layers). More DNA damage means more stress signals. More stress signals means wrinkle-forming enzymes are released and pigment is deposited. And so the cycle continues.

Your crow's feet and age spots aren't the result of that one long weekend at the beach where you turned as red as a lobster. Every moment in the sun, from dawn to dusk, every day and every month and every year, even if it doesn't cause a sunburn or bring on a tan, adds up and damages our DNA.

IMMUNE SUPPRESSION

What has only recently been understood by photobiologists is the surprising fact that the DNA damaged by UV rays also impairs the immune system. This is *not* good news!

Sunlight causes specialized immune cells in the epidermis, the Langerhans cells, to flee the immediate area for up to a week. The cytokines released by the damaged skin cells then cool off the aggressive nature of any remaining white blood cells in the skin and actually make them tolerant to the unfamiliar new substances they encounter. This means your immune system is working at subpar performance.

Some scientists think this may be a way of preventing the immune system from having an allergic response to its own wounded skin. Another theory is that immune suppression is an unintended consequence of the release of so many different signaling molecules with so many messages, not unlike the confusion that reigns when everyone in a room is talking all at once.

As a result of this immune suppression, however, your skin is left vulnerable to foreign invaders, such as bacteria and viruses. And it's unable to respond properly to rogue cancer cells. Pioneering work by the late Dr. J. Wayne Streilein, the Charles L. Schepens Professor of Ophthalmology and professor of dermatology at Harvard Medical School before his death in 2004, showed that people with skin cancer are more easily immune-suppressed than those who have never had skin cancer. And remember, UV exposure that doesn't produce a sunburn can still cripple the immune system for several days.

Bottom line: Sunlight, even without a sunburn, suppresses the immune system so the body is less able to fight off skin cancer and photoaging.

Are you ready for your sunscreen yet?

A BRIEF HISTORY OF SUN PROTECTION

For centuries, the mark left by the sun on unprotected skin was a sign of social status. Lowly laborers who worked outdoors had tanned and photoaged skin, while the elite led an indoor life of leisure and remained pale and undamaged. Proper ladies in the nineteenth century had few worries about photoaging, even though sunscreens as we know them did not yet exist. During the Victorian and Edwardian eras, high bodices, long sleeves, long skirts, hats, gloves, and parasols were a must. Modesty was the driving force in daytime couture, even at the beach, where men and women encased themselves in head-to-toe bathing costumes. Face powders reinforced this image by using poisonous arsenic or lead to blanch the skin. Some women even went to the extreme of painting blue lines on their bosoms to create the effect of skin so translucent that their veins were showing through!

Even before the turn of the twentieth century, fashion and beauty started undergoing a phenomenal shift. Thanks to a widespread fitness craze that took hold in the 1880s—cycling, tennis, golf, cricket, and gymnastics all became fads—clothing gradually became less constraining. By 1910, women's dresses were becoming shorter, more functional, and less bulky. In the years just following the First World War, Coco Chanel arrived in Paris from the seaside resort of Deauville sporting a tan. Chanel envisioned a lifestyle outdoors—complete with beach vacations and open-air sports. Not only did she codify the new ease and make sportswear items chic, but she also cleverly turned the suntan into a clothing accessory—and at the very moment in time when more and more skin on the arms, legs, collarbone, and décolletage was becoming visible. From the short, sleeveless flapper dress of the 1920s, it would take just a few generations and revamped social mores to reach the bikini (1940s), short shorts (1950s), and the miniskirt (1960s).

While fashion changed from the cover-it-up to the let-it-all-hang-out, skin care did not keep up. Instead, we've inherited a legacy of cosmetic calamities resulting from baring massive amounts of unprotected skin to the sun's powerful rays.

While silver UV reflectors and iodine-tinged baby oil, relics of the 1950s and 1960s, are mercifully no longer in style, the allure of the tan is still shockingly potent—especially alarming given the skyrocketing rates of skin cancer. It's no coincidence that this tan-centric lifestyle brings with it an obsession with aging and a crying need to fight its number one cause: overexposure to the sun.

SUNSCREEN BASICS

THE EARLIEST SUNSCREENS

Sun protection is not a new idea. The first sunburn cream to foster recovery from too much baking at the beach was formulated in the 1930s by Milton Blake, an Australian chemist who founded Hamilton Laboratories, a pharmaceutical manufacturing company, to market his discovery. With its sizable population of fair-skinned Celts and Anglo-Saxons, Australia has been at the forefront of sun-care cosmetics ever since. Ambre Solaire, a true UV sunscreen, was created in 1936 by the French chemist Eugène Schueller, one of the founders of L'Oréal. Sunscreens were desperately needed during World War II, when Caucasian soldiers were severely sunburned after spending long days outdoors in the war theaters of North Africa, the Middle East, and tropical Asia.

But outside the needs of soldiers broiling in the sun, the emphasis remained on tanning—not sunburn protection. In 1944, a Florida pharmacist by the name of Benjamin Green invented a suntan lotion that came to be known as Coppertone. Its unforgettable ads showed a pesky dog pulling down a tanned little girl's bathing suit, exposing her milky white bottom. The clear implication was that Coppertone could give you glowing, golden skin, even if your natural skin was as white as a ghost's. It was not until the last quarter of the twentieth century that true sunscreens, designed to prevent sunburn, came into widespread use and began to replace suntan-promoting lotions.

The first widely used sunscreens contained a chemical filter called PABA, which often caused an irritating skin reaction and has since largely been replaced with less irritating chemicals. These sunscreens are based on substances that absorb UV light before it reaches into the skin and diffuse it as harmless heat.

Soon, small metallic particles made of zinc or titanium were developed to make sunscreens even more effective. These particles reflect light away from the skin like a mirror. Unfortunately, they also bounce back some visible light, which makes them appear white on the skin, and it often takes quite a bit of rubbing to disperse the zinc or titanium so that they don't leave a visible film, called ghosting, especially on those with darker skin hues.

Products containing these microparticles are termed "broad spectrum" sunscreens because they protect against UVB as well as UVA rays.

THE SUN PROTECTION FACTOR (SPF)

All sunscreens, whether made in the United States or abroad, are rated by their sun protection factor, or SPF. When you use a sunscreen under ideal conditions, the SPF number indicates how much longer than usual you can stay in the sun without getting sunburned. For example, if you normally can stay in the sun unprotected for twenty minutes before your skin begins to burn, SPF 15 allows you to remain in the sun for fifteen times longer, or five hours, without burning.

But remember: Using a sunscreen, even with a high SPF, does not guarantee that you won't get burned. Let's say you put on an SPF 15 at a beach in St. Croix at 9:00 a.m. and spend a lovely day there, leaving at 3:00 p.m. Well, you will likely be paying the price later, because you were out longer than five hours. Even under ideal conditions, sunscreens reduce, but do not eliminate, sun exposure.

One serious criticism of SPF is that it encourages people to stay out in the sun longer because they feel safe and therefore may get more total sun. A careful study of sunbathers, however, showed they don't stay out any longer when they use a high SPF. At any rate, among similar people the use of sunscreens is related to reduced, not increased, skin cancer risk.

For everyday use against incidental sun exposure in temperate climates, such as driving to work or taking the kids to school, SPF 15 is usually fine. However, if you are outdoors for the better part of the day, SPF 30 is better. In addition, if you have any risk factors for sun damage or skin cancer, such as light-colored eyes, a fair complexion, or a personal or family history of skin cancer, you should use a sunscreen with an SPF higher than 30.

Sunscreens made abroad, with an SPF of 40, 60, or 80 do have a place in a sun-protection arsenal, particularly for those with very fair skin or those going to a tropical beach for a winter vacation after months with little sun exposure. The actual SPF of a sunscreen product as applied by the typical consumer is well below the number on the bottle. It's always better to use a higher number to ensure you get the proper protection.

During the 1980s, competition surged for higher and higher SPF numbers, until the FDA put a lid on it. Inexplicably, instead of helping consumers by making sunscreen labeling as clear as possible, the FDA is *secretive* about regulating SPF numbers. In Europe and elsewhere in the world, sunscreens can be rated with an SPF of 40 or 60; in America, the FDA tentatively ruled that these higher-protection products can only be designated as "30+." (That rule may now be changing—see "This Just In" on page 132.)

As a result of this confusion, some consumers have the impression that high-SPF sunscreens are somehow harmful. In fact, a law firm in California recently filed a class-action lawsuit against sunscreen manufacturers, claiming that they misrepresented their photoprotection. This is absolutely not the case. It is true that some of the high-SPF sunscreens can feel tacky to the touch because the very high percentage of ingredients needed to achieve a high SPF can be sticky. This means people don't often use them the way they are supposed to and they sometimes get burned. However, there is no evidence from any human studies that these ingredients can cause any disease or pose a serious health risk. On the contrary, we know with the utmost certainty that sun exposure damages skin. So when weighing the benefits against the risks, using a higher level of SPF is positively a no-brainer.

Bottom line: SPF measures how long you can stay in the sun without getting a sunburn, and sunscreens also protect you even before you get a burn. But too much sun can overwhelm them and burn your skin badly. There is no credible evidence that sunscreens are harmful.

THE BEST SUNSCREENS

Manufacturers have made continual improvements in their products by screening out a broader range of sunlight that now includes UVA. Sunscreens that reduce both UVB and UVA are called "broad spectrum," but unfortunately, nobody can agree on the way to measure them to compare which ones are better. So we are stuck for now with the SPF rating, which really only measures UVB, and looking for the words "broad spectrum" on the label. (But this too may change; see page 132.)

Remember, no one sunscreen is right for everyone. Some people are allergic to one or the other ingredients, and each person has a preference for texture, how a product rubs or sprays onto skin, what color it leaves behind (if any), and its cost. Some products offer extra benefits because of special additional ingredients that justify a higher price. Keep trying to find one you like and stick with it!

Effective Sunscreen Ingredients

Looking at a sunscreen label can leave you reeling, as many of the ingredients have long, complicated chemical names. This list will help you find the best sunscreen for your needs.

The three most widely used broad-spectrum ingredients (those that protect against UVA and UVB) are

Parsol 1789 or **avobenzone.** Parsol 1789 is a synthetic chemical. It must be carefully formulated with oxybenzone, another synthetic chemical, to prevent it from degrading in sunlight. Neutrogena's Helioplex is a new sunscreen ingredient that incorporates both avobenzone and oxybenzone in one little ball of protection.

Zinc oxide and **titanium dioxide.** These inorganic (or mineral) compounds reflect light away from the skin. Zinc oxide is becoming more popular than titanium dioxide because it is slightly better at absorbing UVA and it leaves less of a white film on the skin when applied.

You also want to look for strong UVB protectants such as ensulizole octyl methoxycinnamate, octisalate (aka octyl salicylate), octylcrylene, or octinoxate. Ideally, your sunscreen should offer one of these along with a broad-spectrum protectant.

RECOMMENDED SUNSCREENS WITH AVOBENZONE PLUS OCTISALATE OR OCTYLCRYLENE

- Coppertone Endless Summer Ultrasheer Sunscreen SPF 15
- DERMAdoctor Body Guard Exquisitely Light SPF 30
- Estée Lauder Multi-Protection Sun Lotion for Body SPF 30
- Hawaiian Tropic Ozone Sport Sunblock SPF 60+
- Kiehl's Vital Sun Protection All-Sport Year-Round Face & Body Spray SPF 25
- La Roche–Posay Biomedic Facial Shield SPF 30
- Neutrogena Age Shield Sunblock with Helioplex SPF 45
- Neutrogena Healthy Defense Oil-Free Sunblock Spray SPF 30
- PCA Skin for Men Total Defense Calming Hydrator SPF 25
- Remergent A.M. Moisture SPF 15 Sunscreen
- RoC Age Diminishing Daily Moisturizer SPF 15

RECOMMENDED SUNSCREENS WITH TITANIUM DIOXIDE AND/OR ZINC OXIDE PLUS OCTINOXATE

- Blue Lizard Australian Suncream—Regular SPF 30+
- Cellex-C Sun Care SPF 30+
- Eucerin Dry Skin Therapy Facial Moisturizing Lotion SPF 25
- M.D. Forté Environmental Protection Cream SPF 30
- Remergent High Intensity SPF 30 Sunscreen
- Shiseido Ultimate Sun Protection Lotion SPF 55
- SunSmart Maximum Protection SPF 30 Lotion

Sunscreens with Mexoryl

The sunscreens available in the United States are not as good as those found in the rest of the world because we have been slow to approve the newest technology with the best sunscreen compounds. One of the best ingredients, Mexoryl SX (ecamsule), was only just recently allowed, and then only in products with SPF 15 or 20. Others have yet to be permitted here. Mexoryl SX combines easily with other compounds, so sunscreen formulas that include it smell better, rub into the skin more easily, and are more easily absorbed, too. In addition, Mexoryl sunscreens do not degrade as easily in sunlight as the others, so they're more effective once you're outdoors. (The products with SPF over 20 may be purchased while traveling abroad and brought back for personal use.)

- La Roche–Posay Anthelios SX Daily Moisturizing Cream SPF 15
- La Roche–Posay Anthelios XL Lait SPF 60
- Lancôme UV Expert SPF 20
- L'Oréal Solar Expertise 50+

Sunscreens with Tinosorb

Tinosorb comes in two formulations, Tinosorb S (bemotrizinol) and Tinosorb M (bisoctrizole), based on new breakthroughs in chemistry. They absorb UV radiation through a stable organic molecule, and their microfine structure allows for both light reflection and light scattering.

Unfortunately, Tinosorb is not yet available in the United States. In March of 2006, more than four hundred pounds of documents were delivered to the FDA in support of its approval. In the next year or so, look for

- Bioderma Spot SPF 100
- Ducray Gel-Crème SPF 15, 30, or 50+

On a positive note, Tinosorb has also been blended into several laundry detergents and fabric softeners, such as Rit SunGuard, which are FDA approved and available in the United States as well as Europe and Australia. When used as directed, it has a cumulative effect on

Sunscreen Ingredients to Avoid

Some individuals have reactions to particular sunscreen ingredients. While that well-known offender PABA has largely disappeared from the marketplace, other common offenders known to cause reactions include padimate A (amyl-p-dimethylaminobenzoate), fragrances, and heavy occlusive oils such as coconut oil.

If you develop a sunscreen reaction, take the bottle with you when you need to purchase a new brand and compare labels. That way you can try to eliminate whatever irritant has caused the problem until you find a sunscreen that works for your skin.

Recently, a Web site with a safety review of sunscreens was set up (www.cosmeticsdatabase.com/special/sunscreens). The ratings may be helpful in separating out the more than 800 brands available, but many of the concerns are overblown and should not scare anyone into avoiding sunscreen use.

clothing. For example, a T-shirt's initial SPF of 8 can be raised to 15 after five washes and to 30 after ten washes.

HOW TO USE SUNSCREEN CORRECTLY

You bought your sunscreen, and you're determined not to get fried on your beach vacation. Much to your surprise and disappointment, that new bottle didn't do what it was supposed to do, and after your very first afternoon on the beach, you ended up spending a miserable night in pain. What went wrong?

Simple: the basic problem almost everyone has with relying on SPF to determine sun protection is that they don't know how much sunscreen to use in order to get that precise SPF. For a sunscreen to have an accurate rating—you put on a 30+ product and want it to act like one!—it *must* be applied in a thick layer. When was the last time you did that?

This Just In: FDA Changes Rules for Sunscreens

Every twenty years or so the FDA tinkers with the sunscreen regulations, and just as this book went to press they issued new rules that will go into effect over the next two years. The first set of changes narrows the SPF rating system found on all sunscreen bottles to refer only to "sun*burn* protection factor" against UVB, rather than broad protection against "sun." The rules also increase the maximum allowable SPF rating from 30+ to 50+. These regulations acknowledge for the first time that there are many other effects of sun exposure beyond sunburn—such as immune suppression and photoaging—and that the SPF rating doesn't necessarily tell you anything about protection from these other dangers. As a result of these rules, new sunscreen labels must also contain a surgeon general–type warning telling consumers to limit sun exposure for their health.

The second set of changes introduces a new rating system for protection beyond sunburn and UVB. A new UVA-defense ranking will appear on the label, with one star meaning little protection against UVA and four stars meaning the highest protection. If a sunscreen does not meet the minimum standard for reducing UVA, it must say so clearly on the label.

Finally, the new manufacturing rules now permit combinations of sunscreens that were previously prohibited such as an organic sunscreen (avobenzone) with an inorganic one (zinc oxide), or avobenzone with ensulizole, and this should pave the way for more pleasing sunscreen formulas that rub on more easily, absorb quickly, and are stable for the whole day.

According to Darrell S. Rigel, clinical professor at New York University's Ronald O. Perelman Department of Dermatology, in order to get an SPF that matches what's on the bottle, you need a full *tablespoon* of sunscreen for your face alone. (Go to the kitchen drawer and measure it out to see how much that is, so you're able to eyeball it. It's a *lot* more than you're used to.) To cover your body, you need one and a half fluid ounces, or a jigger's worth of sunscreen. This can be measured by pumping out two finger lengths of sunscreen.

These amounts are what's used in sunscreen testing, which means that if you don't use the same amount, you will never be getting an accurate SPF. Subjects in controlled clinical studies used less than half the FDA-recommended amount of sunscreen. This means that they got less than half the SPF value that they expected.

Given that most people get only a small fraction of the protection they think they're getting, SPF numbers don't add up to much in practice. It's a little like the mileage sticker on a new car—"actual mileage may vary." In addition, sunscreens with zinc oxide and/or titanium dioxide are often greasier than those with the organic sunscreens, due to the fact that the solvent used to suspend them has an oily feel. They are also difficult to blend in completely in order to avoid the white streaks and the ghosting look. As a result, people tend to rub on only what they can easily blend in and then give up.

And let's not forget that some areas on the body, such as the temples, the ears, and the back, are routinely missed, so in those places the SPF is essentially zero.

Bottom line: To get the full protection of sunscreens, you have to put on about twice as much as you are used to. If you can't do that, consider using a sunscreen with an SPF twice what you usually use and reapply it more often—or, frankly, stay out of the sun.

HOW OFTEN TO REAPPLY SUNSCREEN

Sunscreen should be reapplied every two hours, or immediately after swimming or perspiring.

Remember: Most sunscreens degrade in sunlight. This means they become less effective over time.

One important point is that the organic sunscreens (such as those with avobenzone) take time to start working. You must apply them at least ten to thirty minutes prior to going outside or you'll be protected with SPF 0 when you walk out the door. Be sure to check the active ingredient label on your sunscreen and allow the organics to sink in and get activated before you step outside. Mineral sunscreens with zinc oxide and/or titanium dioxide, however, offer instantaneous protection.

If you use a moisturizer along with a sunscreen, the rule to remember is that sunscreens are applied last. They should be the first product

> ## Don't Use the Same Sunscreen for More than Two Years
>
> Here's something else to think about: sunscreens expire. Most last two years. Of course, if you're using sunscreen correctly, this will never be a problem, but you certainly don't want to pay for a bottle that's been sitting around in a drugstore for more than two years. Companies must put expiration dates on their bottles, and you should use the sunscreen up long before the expiration date approaches.

that encounters the sun's rays, so it's better if they're not obscured or interfered with by other cosmetics.

For those who have a problem applying sunscreen, there are sprays that make it a snap. Especially good are the bottles with a fine spray, as they are quick to apply and are particularly useful when it comes to covering children who are in constant motion. They're also helpful for men who are thinning at the top but still have a little hair; they can find it difficult to rub a cream onto their scalps. This is very important since the top of a man's balding head is a very common area for skin precancers and cancers to develop.

Be aware, though, that it's virtually impossible to achieve the recommended SPF on skin simply by spraying, so use clothing to cover up arms and legs, wear hats with four-inch brims to shield your face, and reapply the sunscreen often.

Bottom line: Apply sunscreens from recently opened bottles after moisturizer but before you go out. Remember to reapply.

RECOMMENDED SPRAY SUNSCREENS

- Clinique Sun-Care Body Spray SPF 30
- Coppertone Continuous Spray SPF 30 product line
- Kiehl's Vital Sun Protection All-Sport Year-Round Face & Body Spray SPF 25

- Neutrogena Fresh Cooling Body Mist Sunblock SPF 30 (best for kids)
- Neutrogena Healthy Defense Oil-Free Sunblock Spray SPF 30
- Vichy Capital Soleil Spray SPF 30 product line

OTHER FORMS OF SUN PROTECTION

Australia has the world's highest rates of skin cancer. That country faces the greatest challenges with sun exposure, as many citizens' ancestors are from England and Ireland and have very fair skin, and they now live an outdoor life on a continent near the equator.

Not surprisingly, Australian scientists have led the way in developing public health programs on sun protection. They may have developed the world's first sunscreen, but they place much less emphasis on sunscreen use than we do in the United States. Instead, they put the highest priority on hats to cover exposed heads and necks and clothing to cover exposed skin on the rest of the body.

Of course, it's not practical or realistic to wear heavy, darkly opaque clothing on hot, humid days. But clothing will always offer protection that doesn't wash or sweat off. You don't have to worry about how much cream you're applying or when to put it on.

Clothing's effectiveness at blocking the sun's rays is measured by a UV protective factor scale. A lightly woven white or pastel T-shirt, for instance, has an SPF factor of about 7; a dark T-shirt ranks in the 10–12 range, and a dark-colored, tightly woven denim shirt can offer protection as high as 1,700. To get a quick estimate of the protection, hold a piece of fabric up to the light. The tighter the weave, the higher the SPF. If you see any pinpricks of light, the weave is loose and the SPF is low.

There are also companies that make clothing and hats with a high SPF factor from the weave of a special lightweight fabric. One of the best known is Solumbra. And don't forget to add Tinosorb (such as Rit SunGuard) to the wash.

When it comes to headwear, save baseball caps for night games. They offer only very limited protection to the forehead, eyes, and nose. This is better than nothing, since one-third of skin cancers occur on the nose, but a baseball cap does nothing for the lower face, ears, or the back of the neck. You should aim for a hat with a brim at least four inches all the way around. Schoolchildren in Australia wear baseball-type hats with Foreign Legion–style flaps covering the ears and the back of the neck.

It is also important to know when to stay out of the sun altogether. The sun's rays are strongest between 10:00 a.m. and 2:00 p.m. Finding shade is a must during the heat of the day. Umbrellas, canopies, and awnings are popular in Australia. So are indoor shopping arcades.

Once you get into the habit of using protective clothing and hats, as well as avoiding the sun in the middle of the day, you can get much more protection than by using sunscreen alone. Australian health officials put sunscreen at the bottom of their list of protection steps, because they don't want the cost of sunscreens to be a factor in deciding about UV protection.

Bottom line: Clothing and hats are also very important ways to protect against the sun.

THE MISUSE OF SUNSCREENS

If you follow these guidelines, a typical five-ounce tube of sunscreen should get used up in a weekend of outdoor recreation. This is not an inexpensive proposition. But it means that sunscreen, regardless of weather or season, should be regarded as something as essential as toothpaste—only a lot more pricey.

On the other hand, paying for skin cancer treatments and bearing its scars is a lot more expensive—and painful.

Still, getting people to use *any* sunscreen is a very serious problem. Most consumers only really think about them during vacations or while playing golf—in essence, only for outdoor play. But studies of the way people actually live their lives show that they get a substantial amount of sun exposure from regular, everyday activities. It's been estimated that up to 80 percent of sun exposure is inadvertent, occurring during our daily comings and goings—the ten-minute errand to town that becomes an hour of strolling from store to store, or the unexpected conversation on the street corner, or getting stuck in traffic on a hot sunny day. Even if you used a sunscreen rigorously during outdoor play, more than two-thirds of your regular, total sun exposure would be missed, leaving you vulnerable to UV assault.

Even worse, many people, especially children and teenagers, don't use any sunscreen at all. A recent survey of NCAA soccer and cross-country teams at four universities, which were composed of educated young men and women spending large amounts of time outdoors, found that a whopping 85 percent reported no sunscreen use in the week before the survey. The study estimated that this is a fairly good representation of the habits of the 250,000 college athletes who participate in outdoor sports each year, as well as other college students.

Let me emphasize one of the most important points of all: Many molecular and clinical studies have shown that the wrinkling and hyperpigmentation of photoaging are not caused just by childhood or teenage sun exposure. In fact, the opposite is true. Recently, research has shown that we get about as much total sun exposure as adults as we did as children and teenagers. (Many men over forty even get *more* sun exposure!) In the well-intentioned pursuit of better sun protection in children, however, some dermatologists and healthcare professionals continue to spread the myth that 80 percent of our lifetime sun exposure occurs *before* the age of eighteen. And it's simply not true!

Here's why clearing up this misperception is so crucial. In order to persist, photoaging needs "upkeep." This means continued and continual UV exposure after age twenty, thirty, and beyond. So as long as you're sticking your face in the sun, the gang of signaling molecules stays active and the cycle of microscarring keeps on spinning. Translation: you are literally causing more wrinkles, sagging, and spots every single time you go out in the sun unprotected.

But if you take care to avoid intense sun, wear hats and protective clothing, and use a sunscreen *no matter what your age,* you will be giving your skin the desperately needed chance to reverse sun damage and prevent precancers and skin cancers.

The Vitamin D Fallacy

Sunscreens have also been tarnished with the highly publicized claim that they cause vitamin D deficiency. Vitamin D is manufactured in the body when UV rays in sunlight react with a chemical in the skin. This vitamin is essential for maintaining the proper level of calcium and phosphorus in the blood and is also vital for keeping bones strong. Too much vitamin D is toxic, so the skin shuts down its production after just five to ten minutes of sunning. Too little vitamin D causes a bone disease called rickets; bones in the leg become brittle and are literally bent into bows by the leg muscles. And vitamin D helps prevent osteoporosis, which is the thinning of bones, especially in postmenopausal women.

Most of us in the medical and scientific community who have seen the studies believe this concern that sunscreens stop vitamin D production is overblown. But we know that the newspaper reports can be confusing, even misleading. Very high doses of vitamin D protect cells against UV rays in the laboratory, but these amounts are toxic and can't be reached in human skin. In fact, not all doctors agree on the right level of vitamin D that should be in the blood for good health—a few even think that Hawaiians living under their tropical sun don't have enough!

What is clear is that you don't need to chuck your sunscreen to get your vitamin D. Doctors are now recommending you get about 800 international units (IU) of vitamin D daily. Most people, especially children, routinely ingest that amount of vitamin D from fortified milk, saltwater fish, and egg yolks, which do not require any light exposure to be active. You should also take a daily vitamin supplement with 800 IU of vitamin D. (Don't worry about getting sick—these amounts are well below a toxic dose.) And as for those who don't drink milk or take vitamins, exposure to only five minutes of sunlight daily, and only to specific body parts, such as the hands or ankles, is all that is needed to maintain stores of vitamin D in your body, even for the elderly. People with darker skin need more time; up to twenty minutes, but never enough to burn. It's far better to take a pill than indulge in unprotected sun worship just to get more vitamin D.

So don't give up and tell yourself that it's too late to bother with sunscreen. Saying things like "The wrinkles are there already, so why bother?" is the absolute *wrong* thing to do! It's when wrinkles are forming that you actually need the most sun protection.

SUN PROTECTION AND THE NEW
SKIN-CARE REVOLUTION

We're only beginning to fight the war against photoaging and skin damage, but there are exciting new products on the market that can help.

DNA repair enzymes are the core of the New Skin-Care Revolution's sun protection formulas, with new products using the advances of molecular biology to optimize the skin's own natural defenses to protect the cells' vital genetic material. The results can be seen in skin in many ways: you'll be less likely to burn, your immune system won't have a meltdown after too much time in the sun, and if you do get sunburned, it won't last as long or peel as much. If you use these new products during the summer months, you can expect smoother skin with fewer lines and wrinkles than if you just use a sunscreen.

This means that the consequences of sun exposure can be avoided, repaired, and reversed. In other words: **It's never too late to repair your skin.**

Let's take a look in greater detail at what works.

DNA REPAIR

The most promising new products in sun protection are those that optimize DNA repair.

As I described before, we're all born with a system of DNA repair enzymes that leaps into action each day to clear our skin of the latest damage. The first enzyme complex searches for the damage and then goes to work, making a nick in the DNA on each side of the damage. These enzymes are then replaced by another set that pries off the short stretch of

DNA containing the damage, leaving the undamaged sections exposed. Right after that, a special enzyme that copies the DNA jumps onto the exposed part and patches the gap. This repair activity takes all of thirty seconds. That's good news, because the enzymes have to patch about 100,000 fused rungs in each skin cell after a day of mild sun exposure at the beach! The bad news is that only half of the needed repairs can be done in one day. And let's not forget that about once in every million patches when there's a mistake that changes the genetic code.

The goal of these new skin-care products is to speed up the natural removal of damage from the skin's DNA. They fight photoaging by stopping the stress signals that set loose the destructive collagen-digesting enzymes (cytokines) and by protecting the immune system.

My lab first realized we were on to something when we were researching topical prescription drugs that could prevent skin cancer. We soon figured out that certain botanical extracts—those with DNA repair enzyme activity—could also be used to tackle photoaging.

These extracts are encapsulated in what we call **liposomes,** a special delivery vehicle uniquely engineered for this purpose. Liposomes are a fantastic advance in skin-care science. The purified DNA repair enzyme may sound like a great technical advance—and it is—but the real breakthrough comes from our being able to deposit the enzyme precisely where it needs to go into the skin.

A liposome is a microscopic balloon made up of an oily lipid membrane, similar in structure to the membranes of skin cells. The DNA repair enzyme is enveloped within the lipid membrane. The size, shape, and electric charge on the liposome membrane allow it to penetrate through the uppermost layers of the skin down to the lower layers, where it can then be absorbed into the living cells.

Once inside the cell, the liposome pops open and releases its enzymes. There, the enzymes seek out the damaged sections of DNA and begin the repair process. It takes about an hour after application for the enzymes to reach their target, the cell's DNA.

It's important to understand why liposomes are such an integral part of DNA repair products. Without them, no cream can truly be effective, as active DNA is only found in living skin cells in the lower layers, not the dead skin cells on the surface.

Bottom line: DNA repair is a natural process that removes the sun damage from skin's DNA. Products that claim to stimulate DNA repair must be able to deliver to where the DNA is—such as by encasing the active ingredients inside liposomes.

Dimericine

Dimericine, developed in my laboratory at AGI Dermatics, is one of the new products that delivers DNA repair enzymes to the skin. The beauty press has already nicknamed Dimericine the "morning-after cream" because it corrects damage and protects skin even after sun exposure.

Dimericine has at its heart a DNA repair enzyme called T4 endonuclease V. This enzyme amazingly seeks out damage in DNA like a laser-guided missile and strikes at the site by cutting out the damaged part of the strand of the DNA. This then signals other repair enzymes to fill in the spot and patch the DNA.

In biochemical parlance, this first step is called the "rate-limiting step," sort of like a bottleneck in an assembly line. Once the bottleneck widens, the whole process of repair can speed up.

Dimericine was first tested on patients with a rare and terrible disease called xeroderma pigmentosum, or XP. Due to a defective gene dealing with DNA repair, XP patients cannot produce all the enzyme components necessary for removing DNA damage. Starting at birth, these patients are extremely sensitive to sunlight, and as babies, many develop painful blisters from even a few moments of sun exposure. Their parents usually take extreme care to protect them during the day and let them play only after dusk—which is why they've been given the poignant moniker "children of the night."

People with XP have skin cancer rates about one thousand times higher than normal, and many die from malignant melanoma before they reach the age of thirty. (To learn more about XP, visit the Xeroderma Pigmentosum Society Web site at www.xps.org.) For our laboratory, undertaking a clinical placebo-controlled, double blind study of Dimericine to help treat such a rare disease was a challenge. It took five years of hard work to recruit thirty XP patients, provide them with lotions for a year, and then follow up their progress for six months.

As we reported in the medical journal *The Lancet* in March 2001,

Dimericine had a dramatic effect on skin cancer in the XP patients. Their rate of new precancerous lesions was reduced by 68 percent compared to the placebo group's. The Dimericine patients also developed 30 percent fewer new skin cancers than the placebo group. Many Dimericine patients reported that their skin felt smoother and more supple. What was also important was that they had no allergic reactions or other significant problems related to the use of Dimericine.

Dimericine is currently being tested in patients who have received kidney transplants. To retain their donated organs, these patients must take immunosuppressive drugs, which have the unwanted side effect of increasing skin cancer risk by a hundredfold. (This problem reinforces the importance of a healthy immune system in protecting the skin against effects of the sun.) We're hoping that Dimericine will also reduce skin cancer in these patients.

Dimericine will be available by prescription once the final clinical studies have been completed and the FDA reviews the results and gives its approval.

Bottom line: Dimericine, while still in the experimental stage, offers the promise of preventing skin cancer by increasing the rate of DNA repair.

Photolyase

Photolyase, one of the enzymes that repairs DNA, has the remarkable ability to bring dead cells back to life! This class of enzymes was discovered accidentally in 1949 when a young graduate student named Albert Kelner forgot to put a plate of yeast back in a dark incubator overnight. The next morning, he discovered that yeast on the plate left out on the table—where it had been exposed to sunlight—survived better than the identical plate put away in the dark. Kelner soon proved that the sunlight had brought the bacteria back to life. He called this "photoreactivation."

Many years later, the DNA repair enzyme responsible for photoreactivation was isolated and named photolyase. Photolyase is an amazing enzyme that has the ability to capture sunlight and channel it to split apart damage-fused DNA, much as photosynthesis enzymes work to capture sunlight to make food for plants. Photolyase is found in many plants and animals, but not in any mammals, including humans.

Photolyase in skin-care products is prepared with the photolyase from the marine plankton *Anacystis nidulans* (listed as "plankton extract" on product package labels). When the enzyme-packed liposomes in these products are applied to the skin in a sunscreen or moisturizer, they are delivered into the skin within one hour of application. Remember, these kinds of products are photoreactive and need some form of light to activate them. About twenty minutes of sunshine or about an hour of indoor light is sufficient to ignite the photolyase enzymes to sweep the DNA clean of most UV damage. Fortunately, photolyase can be activated by light that passes through any sunscreen, so it is an ideal addition to SPF formulas.

What's great about photolyase is that it works very quickly. This makes it an ideal ingredient for skin-care products that you put on in the morning, when your skin is about to be exposed to either daylight or indoor light. Using such products greatly reduces the stress signals that lead to visible signs of photoaging, including sunburn and immune suppression.

Bottom line: Photolyase reverses DNA damage by directly splitting the parts fused together by sunlight.

UV Endonuclease

Other microorganisms have DNA repair enzymes that don't require sunlight activation. These contain an enzyme called UV endonuclease, which stimulates the skin's own natural process of DNA damage removal.

The liposomes in UV endonuclease products are packed with an extract of *Micrococcus luteus* (listed as *Micrococcus* lysate on the product package label), one of the most UV-resistant microbes known to science. This yellowish bug grows everywhere: in soil, in freshwater ponds and brackish seas, even in the frigid waters of the Arctic. In order to survive in these varied but harsh environments, *Micrococcus luteus* has developed a robust DNA repair system to protect its genome.

The liposomes filled with UV endonuclease deliver the DNA repair activity into the skin in a matter of one hour or less. Since they don't require light activation, these products are effective at night as well as during the day.

Many studies have proven the effectiveness of UV endonuclease in activating the skin's DNA repair system. In one study, the enzyme reduced the amount of DNA damage by 76 percent in just twenty-four hours. In another, the cells' immune response remained intact even after sun exposure; in yet another, the horrible after-sunburn flaking and peeling was greatly diminished.

UV endonuclease also has a direct anti-aging effect, acting on the MMP-1 collagen-chomping enzymes that cause wrinkles (for more about MMP-1, see chapter 10).

Bottom line: UV endonuclease increases the normal rate of DNA repair.

RECOMMENDED PRODUCTS FOR DNA REPAIR

- Amway Artistry line
- Avon beComing Un-Flawed Damage Recovery Complex
- ❀ Clinique Stop Signs
- ❀ Estée Lauder Re-Nutriv Ultimate Lifting Creme
- Mary Kay TimeWise Day Solution Sunscreen SPF 25
- ❀ Neways NightScience
- ❀ Neways Rebound After Sun Lotion
- ❀ Nu Skin 180° UV Block Hydrator SPF 18
- Olay Definity Correcting Protective Lotion SPF 15
- ❀ Origins Make A Difference
- ❀ Remergent A.M. Moisturizer SPF 15
- ❀ Remergent DNA Repair Formula
- ❀ Remergent High Intensity SPF 30

Note: The Remergent products are the only ones I know for sure have the right amounts of repair activity.

THE DNA REPAIR BANDWAGON

Since the publication of the first reports on DNA repair, many mystery ingredients have also claimed to increase DNA repair. Are they for real, or are they relying on mystifying scientific jargon to confuse consumers? Let's take a look.

Cat's Claw

Cat's claw (*uña de gato,* or *Uncaria tomentosa*), is a common nutritional supplement made from the bark of a Peruvian creeping vine. It's used as an anti-inflammatory and to boost the immune system, although very few clinical studies have proven it has any real effect when taken orally. Recently it has been promoted to also increase DNA repair, and it's a featured ingredient in the Estée Lauder Re-Nutriv Ultimate Lifting Serum. One publication reported on the laboratory testing of a specially prepared cat's claw extract, but scientists admit they don't know what it is in the extract that might work, and if it does increase DNA repair, they don't know how it does it. Careful here, too, with any old cat's claw because extracts (especially with mystery ingredients) are not standardized and you might not be getting all the effect you expect. The ability of cat's claw to repair DNA is dubious.

Creatine and Folic Acid

Creatine is an important part of muscle and is often taken as a nutritional supplement by bodybuilders. Folic acid (a B vitamin) is also an essential nutrient for cell division, and it is particularly important for pregnant women to have adequate folic acid for their babies. Nivea DNAge Cell Renewal line is designed to deal with damage to the cells' DNA by including these scientific-sounding ingredients. But creatine and folic acid have no particular role in DNA repair other than as essential nutrients for the cell (as does every other vitamin). A particular concern is that folic acid is very sensitive to photodegradation, which means it falls apart when exposed to light on the skin. Whatever the mixture of these two is doing to skin, it is only remotely related to DNA repair. I suggest getting your folic acid requirements from a daily vitamin.

Niacin

Some have claimed that Niacin (vitamin B_3 and its derivatives) can increase DNA repair by being converted into a molecule used by cells to tag the site of damaged DNA, like a bookmark.

The purpose of this bookmark has been a mystery to molecular biologists for many years, yet there is some evidence that a deficit in niacin does inhibit DNA repair. Unfortunately, that doesn't mean that the reverse is true.

Procter & Gamble has reported that Olay Total Effects with VitaNiacin, a form of niacin, improves the color and texture of skin. In addition, the skin-care company Niadyne claims that only its special derivative of niacin, licensed as Niacyl to the Patricia Wexler MD skincare line, sold through Bath & Body Works, is the only form that actually penetrates the skin. That seems unlikely. While niacin does have some moisturizing properties and it may improve your complexion, that's a long way from actually improving DNA repair over the long haul. So look for vitamin B_3 in your skin-care products, but if it's DNA repair you're after, stick to the proven ingredients and products listed here.

Seaweed

The Japanese cosmetic company Kanebo claims that its Sensai Premier The Cream (at $650 a jar!) contains an extract from *Gigartina tenella*, a rare seaweed, that helps repair damaged DNA. However, there is no public information about testing performed on this ingredient and no confirmation from outside the company. Buyer beware.

Selenium

Skin-care products containing the metal selenium also claim to increase DNA repair. Selenium is found in high concentrations in baker's yeast and Brazil nuts, and its consumption has been correlated with reduced rates of certain cancers—but, oddly enough, not skin cancer.

The form of the metal that penetrates into skin is selenomethionine, and the theory is that it activates DNA repair enzyme production at the cellular level. Some laboratory research supports this theory. Despite promising research, however, reliable clinical studies of selenomethionine's effects in human skin have yet to be performed. Selenium is available both in nutritional supplements and in skin-care products, such as the Joli line of tanning products from a company called Glimra. But, yet again, no convincing evidence exists that adding selenium either to the diet or to a skin cream increases DNA repair in human skin.

Care should be taken with selenium. The dosage is very important, since too much selenium can actually damage DNA. In fact, some published studies have shown that instead of reducing cancer, it can actually increase DNA lesions. So proceed with caution.

FIGHTING IMMUNE SUPPRESSION

Because sunlight causes specialized immune cells in the epidermis, called Langerhans cells, to flee the immediate area for up to a week, getting too much sun can leave you with a weakened immune system.

Some oral supplements, such as green tea and vitamins C and E, have shown a small amount of success in protecting the immune system against UV rays. The problem with these nutrients is that whopping doses were used in these studies. It's really hard to drink the equivalent of ten cups of tea or take 5g (e.g., five 1,000-mg pills) of vitamins every day for fifty days. That said, there are two supplements that show some promise in this regard. Look for new products containing aloe and tamarind to be launched in the next few years.

Aloe Vera

Among the new topical ingredients that boost immune function are compounds called oligosaccharides, which are long chains of sugars linked together. Aloe vera gel is a well-known soothing and calming agent, and a preparation of its purified oligosaccharide sugars, called Aloeride, is known to stimulate the immune system. You can easily find large bottles of generic aloe gel in most health food stores, and it's a common ingredient in many skin-care products—but they're notoriously variable in their quality. It's a shame, but not all aloe products are equally effective. Here are some of the good ones:

RECOMMENDED IMMUNE ENHANCERS WITH ALOE

- Clinique After-Sun Balm with Aloe
- Herbalife Herbal Aloe Hand Cream
- Magic of Aloe Nourishing Moisture Lotion
- Optima Organic Aloe Vera Lotion
- Skin MD Natural Dry Skin Care Treatment Shielding Lotion

Tamarind Seed

Another botanical with promise is an extract made from tamarind seeds. The tamarind tree, which grows in Africa and India, has seeds that are commonly used for flavoring sauces. It contains xyloglucans, another type of oligosaccharide that in laboratory studies has been able to protect immune cells from UV rays. Clinical studies on humans have not been completed, but these ingredients appear similar to the successful aloe oligosaccharides.

RECOMMENDED IMMUNE ENHANCERS WITH TAMARIND

- Breathe Delight Multi-Vitamin Hand Cream
- Harmony of Thai Yoghurt Tamarind Body Lotion
- Molton Brown Skinboost 24hr Moisture Mist

PRACTICE SAFE SUN!

Baking in the sun unprotected and getting roasted at the tanning salon won't give you a healthy bronze glow. Instead, they give you prematurely photoaged skin. But you can still enjoy the outdoors if you take reasonable precautions.

■ Find sunscreens with an SPF 15 and an SPF 30 that you like and stick with them.

■ Get in the habit of putting on the SPF 15 sunscreen every morning. Be sure to apply it at least twenty to thirty minutes before going outside.

■ Make one of your mantras "If I don't wear sunscreen every day, I know that I am damaging my skin."

■ Always use a sunscreen with SPF 30 when you expect to have more than a few minutes of casual exposure to the sun. Use as much as you feel comfortable putting on.

■ If your sunscreen bottle is lasting for more than a couple of weeks during the summer, you're not using enough!

■ Don't stop there. When you're outdoors, find shade when you can.

■ Wear hats with broad brims (at least four inches). Get used to having them be a regular part of your wardrobe.

■ Try to wear clothing that has the highest SPF that you can stand. You don't have to wear a sweater when it's broiling hot out, but a dark shirt will give you a lot more protection than a gauzy wrap.

■ Supplement your sun protection, morning and night, with a DNA repair cream.

■ Make another one of your mantras "It's never too early to start protecting myself from photoaging!"

■　■　■

SEVEN

What You Need to Know About Skin Cancer

Despite the constant warnings about needing to protect skin from sun damage, sometimes you'd think that Americans have never heard a word of them. Here are some very scary estimates about sun damage from the American Academy of Dermatology:

- At least 73 million Americans get sunburned each year.

- More than 123 million show the effects of getting too much sun.

- More than 50 million Americans are well on their way to developing some form of skin cancer and already have its precursors: a red, patchy, flaky spot called actinic keratosis (AK).

- More than 1.2 million Americans develop a skin cancer every year, more than all other cancers combined.

These statistics should be more than a wake-up call. They should move you to protect yourself now with an effective skin-care regimen and get you to act at the first signs of trouble.

THE CAUSES OF SKIN CANCER

What we have learned over the last few years is that two things cause skin cancer: the first is a dose of sunlight that changes the DNA in the cells in our skin. The second is ongoing sun exposure that prods the cancer to grow out of control. The second cause is why protection today can stop cancers, even if they were started years ago.

So who gets skin cancer? Among the expected factors is a family history or a personal history of skin cancer—which means some people are just born with a predisposition to the disease. People with light-colored eyes, light-colored hair, and fair skin tend to get more skin cancer than those with darker coloring. The amount of lifetime sun exposure is also a good predictor, and for reasons we don't completely understand, the number of childhood sunburns also increases the risk. (This applies particularly to melanoma, where the *intensity* of the sun, and not the total amount, is most important.)

THE DIFFERENT TYPES OF SKIN CANCER

BASAL CELL CARCINOMA (BCC)

The most common form of skin cancer is basal cell carcinoma (BCC), which appears on the skin as a raised pearly bump or wound with a hard edge that doesn't heal. Fortunately, BCC is not metastatic, and once it's removed, the likelihood of recurrence of that cancer is very low, but it does mean you have an increased risk of getting another BCC somewhere else on your skin.

SQUAMOUS CELL CARCINOMA (SCC)

Squamous cell carcinoma (SCC) is only one-third as common as BCC and is about four times more common in men than women. It is the skin cancer most closely related to total sun exposure. The first sign is often a rough, flaky patch of skin called an actinic keratosis, which can disappear on its own, remain unchanged, or become an SCC. SCCs can also appear as a bump resembling a wart, without starting out as an AK. They are completely curable if caught in time, but left alone they do metastasize and can kill.

MELANOMA

Melanoma is only about one-tenth as frequent as BCC but is the most deadly form of skin cancer. It arises from the pigment-producing cells, and neither BCC nor SCC ever develops into melanoma. It usually appears as a dark but unevenly colored freckle or mole with a ragged edge. Typically, it is asymmetrical—meaning one half is larger or shaped differently than the other half. A melanoma lesion doesn't have to be larger than an eraser at the end of a pencil, or raised above the skin's surface, or even be painful to be deadly. The best defense against melanoma is to catch it early; all suspicious spots should be checked by a dermatologist immediately.

SELF-EXAMINATION

You can also do a self-exam for all types of skin cancer at home—and this can cut your chance of dying from melanoma by more than 50 percent. What you are looking for is a wound, maybe with a hard edge, that doesn't heal; a raised bump with a pearly color; flaky, red patches; or an irregularly shaped or unevenly colored mole.

Assemble two mirrors, a chair, a pencil or a blow-dryer in a well-lit room. To examine the scalp, stand in front of the mirror and run the pencil through a section of hair. Lift the base of the hair shaft up to look at the skin. You can also use a blow-dryer to separate the hair and check the scalp. Start from the bottom and work up. For the back of the head use a second mirror in one hand and the pencil or blow-dryer in the other.

Next, check the head and face, and then move on to the hands (don't forget the nails), elbows, arms, and underarms. Women must also check under their breasts. Use the second mirror to check the back of the neck, upper arms, back, and buttocks. Men need to pay particular attention to the trunk, where their cancer rates are higher.

Then, sit down on the chair and carefully examine the legs—where women must be especially careful because their cancer rates are higher here. Use the second mirror for the back of the legs and don't forget to check between your toes and on the soles of your feet.

TREATING SKIN CANCER

The best way to treat skin cancer is surgical excision, especially a technique called Mohs surgery, which confirms by microscope that the cancer and a margin of healthy tissue around it have been removed. Topical treatment with the drug Efudex is harsh (causing burning red skin) but effective, while the topical drug imiquimod and light therapy are less irritating and are promising improvements. Unfortunately, few effective treatments for melanoma are available if surgical excision doesn't work.

■   ■   ■

EIGHT

Color Changers:
Self-Tanners and Lighteners

The pursuit of beauty has long been fueled by the quest for physical transformation. Nowhere is this quest more poignantly—and more blatantly—expressed than in the desire for a different skin color. Our outer casing is a contradictory flashpoint for human desire, yearning, love, and hate. Skin color unifies cultures into races, and at the same time it serves as a wedge that separates society into leisure and working classes.

These days, no matter what color you are, likely as not you want your skin to be darker or lighter. In Asian countries like Japan, a whopping 40 percent of all cosmetics sold claim to whiten skin. And millions of pale faces in Western countries wish to be bronzed and tanned. Americans and Europeans spend an astonishing $3.2 billion each year on more than 12 million tanning sessions and countless tanning products.

While the Asian preoccupation with alabaster skin reflects centuries-old cultural ideas of beauty, the bronzed-skin esthetic is a relatively recent phenomenon. For centuries in Western countries, darkened or tanned skin signaled outdoor labor, while pale skin meant that you avoided sun with indoor leisure. As soon as women began to join men by the millions working in factories and offices in the twentieth century, that reasoning got turned on its head. Workers became the ones who stayed indoors, toiling and pale, while the upper crust led a leisured outdoor life.

Wars have been waged and centuries of oppression, slavery, and apartheid have been built on little more than the amount of pigmentation in people's skin. No matter what importance we give to skin color, from a genetic standpoint, the differences that divide the races are minute.

DIFFERENCES IN SKIN COLOR

Melanin is the coloring agent found in all animals. In people, it provides color for hair, eyes, and skin. Technically, melanin is amorphous, a globular kind of ink made by specialized cells called melanocytes. They are interspersed among the other cells in the skin, between the upper epidermal layer and the lower dermal layer. Melanocytes are different from other skin cells because they are more closely related to nerve cells.

Skin deep is literally the depth melanin attains—and with good reason. Melanin's main purpose is to absorb the sun's UV radiation. Since skin functions as a barrier to the outside environment, it makes perfect sense that melanin is dispersed near the skin's surface and not planted deep inside.

Each melanocyte is equipped with an enzyme called tyrosinase that produces two different types of pigment: eumelanin, which is black, and pheomelanin, which is red. The relative amount of these pigments, coupled with the size and abundance of the pigment particles, determines skin color for all people, no matter where they live. Within the tremendous range of human skin color, variations can be correlated with climate, geography, and cultural tendencies. Albinos, who exist among all ethnic groups, are completely pale as a result of inheriting from both of their parents a genetic defect in the genes coding for the synthesis of any type of melanin. They have no pigment at all, even in the iris of their eyes, and are extremely susceptible to burns and severe sun damage.

Melanocytes wrap the melanin particles inside little packets called melanosomes and then, borne on the cell's branches, send them out into the surrounding cells at the basement of the epidermis, where they are dispersed. The larger and more numerous the packets, the darker the skin. Eventually, the packets rise to the surface and are shed, so the melanocyte must be working constantly to replenish the melanin and maintain the color. If it falls behind, the skin pales; if it goes into overdrive, the skin develops freckles or darkens.

People fade as they get older—the melanocytes slow down their production of melanin. Women tend to get lighter than men; one hypothesis is that women need more vitamin D from sunlight as they age to strengthen their bones and fight osteoporosis, and less melanin allows for more absorption of the needed light waves.

The melanin residing in the upper skin layer, where it can be shed, is entirely different, by the way, from the permanent color of tattoos. With tattoos, ink is injected through a needle beneath the epidermis, down into the dermis, where there is no migration to the surface. The ink may diffuse sideways, turning that catchy phrase into a barely legible Rorschach blot, but it won't be dispersed entirely. This makes tattoo removal a tough process.

A host of products and procedures are touted to turn skin to a desired shade—either darker or lighter than what naturally exists. Can what's readily available today safely and effectively lighten or darken skin to the exact tone we desire?

VARIATIONS IN SKIN AMONG ETHNIC GROUPS

Skin characteristics among ethnic groups really don't differ as much as you might think. So while anti-aging products have traditionally been developed and marketed to the American mainstream—meaning Caucasians—more and more skin-care specialists are developing makeup and skin-care products for the "ethnic" market. These products are fine-tuned to light but easily tanned Asian skin, darker and easily tanned Hispanic skin, and the darker skin of African Americans and South Asians. Mixed in among these categories are every conceivable shading.

But how justified is this color categorizing? Considering that all 6 billion people alive today share 99.99 percent of their DNA and that we're all descended from a small tribe of people who lived in eastern Africa, the diversity we see today is the result of only about 7,500 generations of descendants from that group.

The problem with making sweeping simplifications about an ethnic group's skin condition is that how they look is greatly influenced by their lifestyles and outdoor habits. The most striking example is among Japanese who move to America. In Japan, there's a high rate of stomach cancer and very low rates of skin cancer. In Hawaii, however, there's a dramatic drop in stomach cancer rates and a huge rise in skin cancer. There is no doubt that these changes have to do with lifestyle.

Both consumers and skin-care professionals have decided opinions about skin differences among ethnic groups, but there are surprisingly few objective scientific measurements of these variations. Some studies suggest that the stratum corneum in black skin may be thicker than others and therefore less likely to become irritated. On the other hand, Asian skin is said to have a thinner stratum corneum, making it more prone to irritation. But there are just too many conflicting reports to allow scientists to be confident about making sweeping generalizations.

One common perception is that Caucasian skin tends to be dry and that oiliness increases with the darkness of skin. Contrary to this assumption, consumer studies show that African Americans and Asians are more likely to use moisturizers than the general population. In fact, objective measurements of basic skin characteristics, such as the strength of the skin's barrier, the amount of water and lipids, and skin acidity, are often conflicting and most show little or no difference among Caucasian, African American, Hispanic, and Asian skin. Ethnic skin-care product lines often feature toners with astringents such as witch hazel and oily or waxy moisturizers containing cocoa butter or shea butter. These may be a beauty choice, but they are no more needed in black skin than in white skin.

The most significant differences among ethnic skin types are photo-sensitivity, discoloration, sensitivity, and scarring. Obviously, the darker the skin tone the more resistant it is to sunburn, and in general there's also less skin cancer. But don't be fooled by these generalizations—for all skin types, sun exposure ages you. It also causes DNA damage, even without a sunburn, and suppresses the immune system.

Bottom line: Contrary to popular belief, aside from a few specific conditions, skin characteristics don't vary much among people of different skin color. Everyone can benefit from increased sunscreen use and the same DNA repair products.

TOO MUCH AND TOO LITTLE COLOR, AND SCARS
The flip side of dark skin having better sun protection is that even a small unevenness in tone is much more readily apparent and can be-

come a chronic problem. When things go really wrong, melanocytes stop making pigment altogether, causing lighter hypopigmentation spots to form. This is called vitiligo, and its seems to be an autoimmune disease, where the body attacks its own melanocytes. It's very difficult to treat with OTC products, so it's best to consult a dermatologist if you have it.

Skin can also become unevenly dark, a condition called melasma. Melasma is common because it's hard for all the melanocytes to coordinate the higher output of melanin and its even distribution. Beyond that, every wound or flare-up of skin also involves a melanocyte response, and changes in melanin output by these cells creates darker hyperpigmentation spots.

The solution is to avoid skin-care regimens that have the risk of irritation or invoke a wound-healing response, such as peels, microdermabrasion, lasers, high concentrations of peroxides, or bleaching agents. Treat irritations or wounds, especially to the face, with moisturizers that contain calming agents like evodia extract or chamomile. Realize that, as we've discussed, many botanicals and fragrances also frequently cause unexpected irritation.

For some reason not yet well understood, the skin of many, but not all, darkly pigmented people easily overreacts to a wound and creates too much collagen. This forms raised scars called keloids. This can be a serious problem and can arise after something as simple as piercing an ear. Once keloids form, there is no known effective treatment, although in some cases injected steroids may shrink them. A promising new therapy is 5 percent imiquimod cream, which only needs to be used once every three or four days for eight weeks. Those who are prone to keloids must be very careful with any skin-care treatments that cut or wound the skin.

And then there are lasers. Many types of lasers are dangerous to dark skin, because more melanin means more light is absorbed, which can burn or trigger keloids. Some of the newer lasers can target problems in darker skin, but you must see an experienced professional with specially selected light sources and extensive experience—or you could wind up with spots of different hues on your face.

Bottom line: Skin of color is more likely to have uneven pigmentation, such as melasma or vitiligo. It is also more likely to respond to wounding with keloids, which are areas of scarring.

THE TRUTH ABOUT TANNING

Tanning began as a fashion trend and then a whole "healthy lifestyle" industry sprang up around it. Just as we once thought smoking was glamorous and now recognize it as a deadly habit, we now understand the dangers of tanning.

THE MYTH OF THE PROTECTIVE TAN

A tan is supposed to be a protection against skin cancer, isn't it?

At first blush, it should be. Dark-skinned Africans have far lower rates of all types of skin cancer than those with lighter skin, even though they tend to live in areas of intense sunlight. But don't be fooled. No tan is ever healthy!

Skin color depends not only on the amount but also on the type of melanin the skin contains. All skin has a mixture of two types of melanin: eumelanin and pheomelanin. Blacks have a predominance of eumelanin; Celts have predominantly pheomelanin. Eumelanin offers more protection from sunlight than pheomelanin, so even though redheads have about half the melanin found in dark skin, they have much less than half the solar defense and more than twice the skin cancer rates. White South Africans have a lifetime risk of skin cancer fifteen times greater than that for black South Africans.

Eumelanin comes in much larger globules than pheomelanin. This means more protection. Both types of pigment are carefully placed by the melanocytes in little "caps" that cover the nuclei of the surrounding cells. This capping gives the greatest protection for DNA, which is tightly packaged inside the nucleus of the cell.

The point here is that your genes—which control the amounts of eumelanin or pheomelanin produced and the size of their pigment packages—determine how much your skin color will protect you from the sun.

The color you get with a tan—whether from the sun, a tanning lamp, or a bottle—just isn't the same, and it doesn't protect your skin very much from UV damage. When melanocytes produce more color after sun exposure, they don't carefully deposit it over the nuclei of the neighboring cells (the way natural melanin positions itself in the skin). Instead, they spew much of it throughout the skin as melanin dust granules. That is why a tan gradually fades as the granules are sloughed off from the surface, along with the usual dead skin cells.

Having a tan is not the same as having naturally dark skin. A tan provides an SPF of only about 4—and comes at the cost of serious DNA damage.

Still, people are literally addicted to tanning. Many of us have felt the sensation of warmth and calm while getting roasted on the beach. We're not just enjoying a relaxing day—the sun causes our bodies to produce endorphins that induce a lovely feeling of euphoria. But while a sunbathing tan might make you feel good, no one should think that natural, parlor, or lotion tanned skin gives you permission to spend unprotected time in the sun!

TANNING PARLOR HYPE

Americans who flock to tanning parlors expose themselves to whopping doses of ultraviolet light, and UV radiation damages the DNA of each skin cell it encounters. The overworked melanocytes react by trying to produce and disperse extra melanin, as if they could pull down the skin's window shade. But this shade takes about ten days to grow in, and in the meantime exposed skin has no protection.

Despite all the tanning-industry hype, the plain fact is that no tanning lamp is safe. Nearly everyone who has ever used a sunlamp has literally been burned at least once, and many get burned repeatedly. One reason is that customers pay for sessions by the length of time they spend under the sunlamp, but since they don't control the lamp, they don't control the amount of UV radiation that they receive.

A review of more than a dozen clinical studies concluded that tanning bed and sunlamp exposure causes a significantly increased risk of malignant melanoma—the deadliest form of skin cancer (see chapter 7). In 2007 congress passed the TAN Act, directing the FDA to consider putting a warning on tanning beds saying that "UV causes skin cancer."

So before you hit the tanning bed, know that the price may include damaged skin, accelerated aging, and increased risk of disease and death.

SUNLESS TANNING

The good news is that if you're still craving that bronzed look but don't want to damage your skin or risk your health to get it, there are safe alternatives to tanning. Sunless tanners are a new cosmetic category that blurs the distinction between makeup and skin care.

SELF-TANNING AT HOME

All self-tanners on the market are based on a chemical called DHA (dihydroacetone), which turns an orange-brown color when it binds to proteins in the skin's top layer. Why not put melanin on the skin itself to create a tan? Well, melanin is not, strictly speaking, a chemical, but various-sized globules of an oily protein pigment. It can't pass through the skin from the top, so DHA is the alternative.

Here are some tips for self-tanning at home:

■ Start early. Give yourself a week or two before the target date. Be prepared to try a few products before you find one you really like, as it's impossible to know exactly which precise color will appear on your skin by reading the product label. Test the self-tanner on a small spot on your inner forearm.

■ Cleanse and exfoliate your skin thoroughly with an AHA exfoliator, then shave your legs before starting. If you wax, wait a day before beginning.

■ To keep a natural look, put a thin film of your favorite moisturizer between your fingers and toes, and around your nails. Don't forget a dab in your belly button.

■ Self-tanners should not be applied too close to the eyes, as they can irritate the delicate tissue there.

■ For liquid self-tanners: Apply from feet to neck, sideways and then up and down. Only dispense a palm-sized amount at a time.

■ For spray self-tanners: Begin in the shower or while standing on a towel. Hold the spray six to eight inches away and start from the feet and move to the neck, using broad strokes.

■ No matter how you apply the self-tanner, use it sparingly around the knees, elbows, and heels, as these areas have particularly thick surface layers that react to form a deeper color than on the rest of the body.

■ Be patient. Wait at least twenty minutes before putting on clothes. Self-tanners take several hours to work. Expect to reapply once or twice more over the following days to achieve an even or darker color. Set reasonable expectations and go for a shade lighter than the one you envision—you'll look better.

■ Don't be disappointed when the tan fades in a few days. Over time, the upper layers of skin that are bound to the DHA will be shed, and the color will fade. Color on the face will fade the fastest. Think of it as body makeup, not an endless tan!

■ Self-tanners that do not contain sunscreen (and most of them don't) do not protect against sunburn or other aging effects of the sun.

RECOMMENDED SELF-TANNERS

- ❀ Clarins Self Tanning Instant Gel
- ❀ Clinique Self-Sun Body Self-Tanning Mist
- Coppertone Endless Summer Sunless Tanning Lotion
- ❀ Dior Bronze Self-Tanner Natural Glow
- ❀ Estée Lauder Sun Performance Self Tan Towelettes
- Neutrogena Instant Bronze Sunless Tanner and Bronzer in One

SELF-TANNING IN THE BRONZING BOOTH
Those who seek a perfect tanning application every time may want to try a private session where they can get help—either from a trained esthetician

in a spa or salon or by one of the automated spray-application systems. A growing number of tanning-bed facilities are finally getting smart about sun damage and are substituting spray units for sunlamps. These systems eliminate much of the guesswork of the at-home self-tanning process and have a reputation for leaving the smoothest, least-orange, most snafu-free tan that can come out of a bottle. But beware: during the process, eyes, nose, and ears must be covered well. To get a natural look, the elbows, knees, and belly button need a lighter touch than the rest of the body.

The best-known salon spray is Mystic Tan Tanning Myst, with DHA and aloe vera. It's dispensed in a booth featuring spray jets that hit the entire body in only ninety seconds. Mystic Tan's electrostatic technology, where clients stand on a metal plate during the spray process, is said to prevent the buildup that causes the orange effect. The resulting tan is instantaneous and is meant to last up to seven days—although frequent tanners say it can turn splotchy.

BRONZING MAKEUP

Another alternative to a tan is bronzing makeup, which is available in a wide variety of shades and textures, in powder, liquid, and gel form, and with or without shimmer. Some formulations can be used all over the face as foundation; others are applied to the cheeks instead of blusher; still others are body makeup for use on the collarbone, décolletage, shoulders, arms, and legs.

The trick with a bronzer is to apply it wherever the sun would hit the skin—over the bridge of the nose, on the cheekbones, at the top and sides of the forehead, on the chin, and on the collarbone. Don't apply too much or you'll just look fake!

RECOMMENDED BRONZING MAKEUP

- Bare Escentuals i.d. bareMinerals All-Over Face Color
- Estée Lauder In the Sun Shimmer Sunscreen SPF 15
- Guerlain Terracotta Fresh Bronzing Gel
- IsaDora Bronzing Powder
- Laura Mercier Bronzing Powder
- Lorac Bronzer

- ✿ Nars Bronzing Powder
- ✿ Tarte Mineral Powder Bronzer
- ✿ Vincent Longo Sole Mio Duo Bronzer

SELF-TANNERS OF THE NEW SKIN-CARE REVOLUTION

The holy grail of tanning would be a technology that safely lets skin produce more of its own natural skin pigment—triggering a truly safe tan. No one ingredient has yet been perfected, but many scientists around the world are hoping to discover and perfect a substance that would not only tan skin naturally, but help protect against skin cancer developing.

DNA Fragments

One approach is to use DNA fragments, which are supposed to resemble sunburned DNA, to trick skin cells into reacting as if they really have been damaged. This would trigger the tanning response. The idea is to coat the skin with a cream containing short pieces of DNA, and it would take about a week to produce a natural tan.

So far, this method seems to work in guinea pigs, but it's still controversial as to whether or not it works in people. Scientists are cautious because it's not clear that a topical application of naked DNA will be able to sink down to living DNA in the epidermis. Frankly, if it were this easy, then gene therapy, or the process of correcting defective DNA with correct DNA, would be much farther along, and we'd be able to cure skin diseases with topical creams.

Melanotan

Another experimental tanning product was uncovered during experiments with an alpha-melanocyte stimulating hormone. After injecting a piece of this hormone under the skin of volunteers, a tan formed near the injection site. The discovery, called Melanotan, is now undergoing clinical trials in Australia and Europe. Melanotan injections nearly doubled skin pigment in fair-skinned individuals, although about one in six patients experienced side effects like nausea or facial flushing serious enough to cause them to quit the trial.

Norbordiol

A synthetic chemical called Norbordiol also shows promise as a natural self-tanning agent. This compound switches on the skin's production of nitric oxide, a key signaling molecule. Melanocytes respond to higher levels of nitric oxide by making more of their own melanin, dispersing it as they do a natural tan. Because it is an oil-soluble chemical and not a peptide, Norbordiol can be rubbed onto the skin and doesn't have to be injected like Melanotan. The resulting tan is mild, and much more study is needed to see if it will truly work as a natural self-tanner.

Note: Because these last two chemicals, Melanotan and Norbordiol, increase nitric oxide, they are being tested in the treatment of erectile dysfunction.

BRIGHTENERS AND LIGHTENERS

In some cultures, a porcelain white complexion is the standard of true beauty. In others, having an even skin tone, free from spots and blotches, is the far more realistic goal. Countless new skin-care products claming to lighten and brighten have been launched to tackle the problem. Those small areas of discoloration called age spots or liver spots, found predominantly on the faces, arms, and hands of light-skinned people, used to be regarded as an inevitable result of growing old. Today, these spots are appearing in people decades before their first senior moment. That is a dangerous sign that sun worship is out of control!

The proper name for these spots is "solar lentigines." A single spot is called a "solar lentigo." They're a direct result of accumulated sun damage, which triggers a nest of melanocytes to lose control and produce too much pigment. By themselves, these spots are not dangerous, although they can be unsightly. Many who are unhappy with their age spots resort to whitening or bleaching products and may finally start using sunscreen religiously. Others are lulled into a false sense of security, and assume that all dark patches are harmless age spots, not realizing that their little dark spots are really melanoma. (For more information on how to distinguish a solar lentigo from a melanoma, see chapter 7. If you have any doubt, see your dermatologist immediately!)

In skin that's been particularly photoaged, usually on forearms or the upper chest, a condition called poikiloderma can appear. This produces dark spots of excessive pigmentation mixed with white spots where all the pigment-producing melanocytes have been killed off and the skin has thinned.

The best treatment for all these spots is prevention. Stay out of the sun, or when you do go outside, always use a sunscreen!

In young adults, age spots range in shade, from light tan to dark brown. In older people, a different lesion, more typically called a liver spot, is made up of clumps of undigested cell debris. This is rolled together and engulfed by a colony of immovable cells into a microscopic junkyard. These liver spots have a distinctive blue tone.

Areas of discoloration also can appear during pregnancy or among those using oral contraceptives; this condition is called chloasma, or the mask of pregnancy. Rapidly changing hormonal levels trigger the wrong signals to melanocytes, sending them into pigmentation panic. (Fortunately, chloasma often goes away after birth or when birth control pills are discontinued, allowing hormones to return to normal levels.) People with medium and darker skin tones often use whitening products to treat patches of melasma and areas of post-inflammatory hyperpigmentation.

TRIED AND TRUE BRIGHTENERS

No lightening treatment is perfect or permanent, and brighteners are the least effective in those with darker skin tones. They also don't work overnight. When you start using one of these products, give it two or three months before deciding it doesn't work, and bear in mind that some ingredients, like hydroquinone or azelaic acid, can be irritating.

Age spots caused by sun exposure respond to spot treatment; colored spots from pregnancy usually fade after birth, so begin with mild treatments and slowly work up to higher strengths. Patches of melasma or general darkening require determination and vigilance, as well as long-term therapy.

In all cases, if you don't use a strong sunscreen, you might as well not bother trying any whitener. You'll just get new spots (and a lot more wrinkles)!

Hydroquinone

For dark spots, the topical treatment of choice is hydroquinone. Its primary function is to inhibit the enzyme tyrosinase, which forms pigment, and it has become the gold standard for skin lightening.

Hydroquinone has been used for decades by millions of people around the world, and its risks and side effects, like those of any drug, are well known. These are usually due to overuse (longer than twelve weeks), when bluish discolorations, called onchronosis, can form. Laboratory studies in cultured cells and animals suggest that hydroquinone can cause mutations in DNA, but an international study group found there was no evidence that it posed a cancer risk in people. Nevertheless, many countries have banned hydroquinone's use in skin-care products. The FDA is also considering restricting its availability.

This is vexing to U.S. dermatologists, almost all of whom have never seen a case of onchronosis in their professional careers and very likely never will (there have only been 15 cases out of 50 million users). In fact, there is not a single confirmed report of cancer due to hydroquinone in the fifty years that it's been on the market. What's more, arbutin, a part of mulberry or bearberry extract that is converted by the body into hydroquinone, is legally used in cosmetics. This makes no sense whatsoever. When hydroquinone attacks tyrosinase, the cell really can't tell whether it came from a fruit or a factory!

Hydroquinone at 2 percent strength is available for now in many OTC products. Here are a few tips for their use:

■ Any hydroquinone product should first be tested on the inside of the elbow overnight for an allergic reaction such as redness or itching.

■ If none appears, go ahead and apply a thin film over the dark spot twice a day. The spot should fade in a few weeks; if you see no results in three months, stop treatment before irritation develops and consult a dermatologist about other options. Stronger concentrations are available by prescription.

▣ Keep your expectations reasonable; these products lighten but don't erase spots, and they are most effective in light-skinned people.

▣ Since hydroquinone is a delicate chemical that easily oxidizes to a brownish color, keep all products tightly closed and away from excessive heat and light.

▣ Any lightening agent leaves the skin more sensitive to sunlight and is labeled with a warning that sun protection is needed. Some lighteners include sunscreens in their formula. But the effectiveness of sunscreens in these formulas is questionable—since a lightener should be applied in a thin layer, the sun protection provided is so marginal it's not even given an SPF number. Be sure to use an SPF 15+ sunscreen on the affected area and avoid the sun wherever possible while using hydroquinone creams.

RECOMMENDED 2 PERCENT HYDROQUINONE CREAMS

- Dr. Jan Adams Women of Color Skin Lightener
- Esotérica Fade Cream Regular
- ☀ Exuviance Essential Skin Lightener Gel
- Porcelana Skin Lightening Serum
- Skin Effects by Dr. Jeffrey Dover Advanced Brightening Complex

ALTERNATE BRIGHTENERS

No other single brightener is as effective as hydroquinone, but if you are sensitive and need an alternative, consider those below. As some of these brighteners can be irritating, always test them on your inner arm, inside the elbow, first. If there's any reaction, such as redness or itching, do not use them!

Azelaic Acid

Another popular lightening ingredient is azelaic acid, found in wheat and barley. It's pretty effective against most types of discolorations, including melasma and solar lentigines. How it works, however, is not all that clear, and since it is only a weak inhibitor of tyrosinase, you need a high concentration (15 percent or more) for it to work. Such high levels can be irritating for some people—a concern for those with darker skin, who can react with postinflammatory hyperpigmentation spots.

RECOMMENDED AZELAIC ACID BRIGHTENERS

* DDF Intensive Holistic Lightener
* Jan Marini Skin Research Factor-A Plus Mask
* Peter Thomas Roth Potent Botanical Skin Brightening Gel Complex

Kojic Acid

At the beginning of the twentieth century, scientists in Japan fermenting malted rice into sake discovered a by-product: kojic acid. We've since learned that kojic acid inhibits the melanin-producing enzyme tyrosinase, making it the first alternative to hydroquinone. It quickly became popular in Japanese skin-care products.

Some clinical studies in Western medical journals support kojic acid's claim for brightening, particularly in melasma, but its use is limited because this ingredient is not particularly stable and high dosages are needed. Like azelaic acid, it too can be irritating, and it often causes allergic reactions and dermatitis. Also test it on a small spot on the inner arm before using it.

RECOMMENDED KOJIC ACID BRIGHTENERS

* GreatSkin Fruit Acid Gel with Kojic Acid 15%
* Neova Kojic Complex Gel
* Reviva Brown Spot Night Gel

Retinoic Acid and Retinol

The vitamin A derivatives retinoic acid and retinol are superstars in the fight against wrinkles, as we will see in chapter 10. Well known for their ability to increase skin-cell turnover, they are added to many lighteners to speed the removal of pigment granules and accelerate the effects of other whitening agents.

Retinoic acid and retinol must be used continuously for best results, but they always make skin thinner and more vulnerable and sensitive to the sun. Always use a sunscreen if you choose a lightener that has retinoic acid or retinol added to it. High-concentration retinol products are ❀ Replenix Retinol Smoothing Serum 10X and ❀ Remergent Advanced Retinol 0.4% or 1.0%.

Vitamin C, Ascorbic Acid, and MAP

One of the most popular skin lightening ingredients is a stabilized derivative of vitamin C called magnesium ascorbyl phosphate, or MAP. Research studies clearly show that MAP inhibits tyrosinase, the main pigment-forming enzyme. But there have been few clinical studies, and many dermatologists who recommend MAP rely on a Japanese study of a 10 percent formula that was tested on a grand total of fifty-nine patients. While more than half the Japanese patients with abnormal pigmentation saw an improvement, only three out of twenty-five people with "normal" skin saw any skin brightening.

Despite this, MAP and other forms of ascorbic acid (vitamin C) remain widely used in skin lightening products. To be effective, they must be formulated in high concentrations (5 percent or greater), as in ❀ DHC White Cream.

A product that combines both retinol and vitamin C for brightening is ❀ EmerginC Multi-Vitamin and Retinol Serum.

NOT QUITE BRIGHTENERS

The enormous demand for skin lightening and brightening has spawned a host of wannabe ingredients and not-worth-the-trouble products. Here is a rundown of what to avoid.

Botanicals

Many plant extracts, such as cucumber seed, grape, hibiscus flower, mulberry, *Rumex occidentalis* (a perennial herb), saxifrage (related to magnolias), and scutellaria (blue skullcap, an herb related to rosemary), may well have skin whitening properties, but their active components are unknown and there's little data to support their use. Some specially prepared extracts no doubt do work, but it's likely because of their other active ingredients, like arbutin, azelaic acid, or kojic acid.

Ultimately, if a brightening product lists a plant extract on its label, it is nearly impossible to know if it's going to do any good without trying it. Look for other ingredients first.

Licorice Root Extract (Glycyrrhizinate)

Licorice root extract, which has a component called glycyrrhizinate, is known to be an anti-inflammatory. Glycyrrhizinate is also a strong inhibitor of tyrosinase, but any published data on whether or not it truly works to lighten skin is scarce. Nevertheless, it's a popular clarifying agent, found in ✺ Godiva Licorice Skin Whitening Cream and ✺ Sothys Blanc Perfect Fluid, both of which also contain the vitamin C lightening agent MAP, and ✺ DermaLite by Beauty Naturally, which also contains kojic acid.

Melatonin

Melatonin is a hormone discovered in 1958 by Dr. Aaron Lerner, a Yale dermatologist. Synthesized in the pineal gland deep inside the brain, it helps regulate sleep patterns. Dr. Lerner first noticed that it lightened the color of frog skin.

Some companies that hype melatonin claim that it can lighten human skin as well. But Dr. Lerner himself tested for this effect in humans and reported in 1977 that he saw no significant lightening benefits. Several studies in people have shown that melatonin provides a modest protection against sunburn, with an SPF of about 2. But in the end, melatonin is not what you need.

BRIGHTENERS OF THE NEW SKIN-CARE REVOLUTION

Recent discoveries about skin and pigment production have greatly improved lighteners. The best of them can more potently inhibit tyrosinase, because they are better at getting the active ingredients into the melanocytes, where they can get to work.

Arbutin

Purified from mulberry or bearberry extract, arbutin became the favored brightening ingredient in Japan after interest in kojic acid faded in recent years. Using arbutin is a clever way to get around the ban on hydroquinone, since this botanical extract is basically the same chemical, but with a sugar molecule attached. Once in contact with the skin, enzymes in the epidermal layer cleave off the sugar and slowly release hydroquinone.

While arbutin takes a few weeks longer to work, it may be just as effective as hydroquinone—but with less risk of irritation.

RECOMMENDED ARBUTIN WHITENERS
* DHC Alpha-Arbutin White Cream
* Shiseido Whitess Intensive Skin Brightener

Ergothioneine

Ergothioneine is an amino acid that humans must get from the grains in our diet. As I mentioned in chapter 5, ergothioneine is an antioxidant, like vitamin C, but it also binds to the trace metals that are essential for tyrosinase to function. When we tested it in our laboratory and in clinical studies, we found that it not only inhibited tyrosinase, but also stopped cells from producing pigment following UV exposure.

RECOMMENDED ERGOTHIONEINE LIGHTENERS

* Cellex-C Advanced-C Eye Firming Cream
* Remergent Clarifying Concentrate[2] (this product and Sepiwhite have the highest concentration of ergothioneine on the market)
* ShiKai Adult Formula Borage Dry Skin Therapy Lotion

Sepiwhite

Sepiwhite is a mixture of natural amino acids with a lipid base to help it penetrate into skin. It is designed to block the signals that turn on pigment production in melanocytes. The evidence shows it has about one-quarter the strength of hydroquinone, but it is also far less irritating.

RECOMMENDED SEPIWHITE PRODUCTS

* Dr. Temt White Serum
* Elizabeth Halen Sepiwhite Lipo-Facial Cream
* Remergent Clarifying Concentrate[2] (also with ergothioneine)

■   ■   ■

NINE

Antioxidants and the Emperor's New Clothes

Vitamin C . . . pomegranate . . . green tea . . . copper . . . idebenone . . . CoQ10. They sound delicious. Or exotic. Or miraculous. Right? *Wrong!*

Whether squeezed from a lemon, plucked from a shrub, extracted from a mine, or mixed in a lab, all of these ingredients claim to be antioxidants—the stuff of skin-rejuvenation hope and promise. As a result, these and many other familiar (and not-so-familiar) antioxidants have found their way into hundreds of different skin-care products. They are *essential,* trumpet the claims, in the fight against the villainous rogue chemicals known as free radicals.

Found naturally in all animal and plants, antioxidants supposedly protect us from future assault and undo the damage that's already been done as well. And there's no denying that a certain pleasure can be taken in thinking that those virtuous antioxidants are busy vanquishing the evil free radicals (generated by sunlight, pollution, and even manufactured by our own bodies) and giving them the heave-ho they deserve. After all, aren't those free radicals to blame for bombarding our skin and causing immediate redness and irritation, gradually leading to deeper wrinkles, sagging skin, mottling, sallowness, and just about every other visible sign of aging? Even cancer?

Enlisting antioxidants in the fight against free radicals has been the most important scientific promise sold to consumers since the 1980s. But fifty years after it was first proposed, the free radical theory as applied to skin aging is still missing serious supporting evidence. In this chaper we'll take a look at whether antioxidants can live up to this hype.

THE EMPEROR'S NEW CLOTHES

Though this is rarely acknowledged in the skin-care world, the science behind the proposition that free radicals cause skin aging and that antioxidants can fix it just doesn't quite add up. Someone needs to ask if this isn't a case of the emperor's new clothes!

In fact, this free radical concept is nothing more than a theory. So I decided to put it to the test. I took a bottle of hydrogen peroxide, which is a concentrated form of oxygen radicals, and spotted it directly, undiluted, onto the skin of my forearm. Now, hydrogen peroxide unleashes the nastiest of free radicals and should be a fair test of what happens when they supposedly attack skin. Hydrogen peroxide is used, of course, to sterilize cuts and scrapes, and when enough of it reaches the nerves it causes pain. But in my case, the skin of my forearm was intact—and it didn't hurt at all.

The treated spot, however, did immediately whiten. This is called a "blanching reaction," meaning the blood vessels deep in my skin contracted. After only a few minutes, the vessels returned to normal, and the white spot disappeared. Surely, I reasoned, if there had been enough hydrogen peroxide to close down the capillaries in my skin, then free radicals must have been waging war in my epidermis, right?

So I waited and waited, yet no redness, no inflammation, and no sunburn formed. In fact, despite the release of a billion-billion (10^{18}) peroxide- and hydroxyl-type oxygen radicals in each drop, nothing happened to my skin. *Nothing*. Certainly not anything that in any way resembled an hour of unprotected sun exposure. I had to ask myself, if free radicals are so dangerous, why didn't I see at least *some* kind of reaction?

And then I had to ask a few more questions. What kind of explanation have the proponents of free radicals given to consumers? Are antioxidants really the single most important treatment for skin aging? Or are they an overblown chemical curiosity put to work by Madison Avenue to sell fruit juice and skin cream?

FREE RADICALS AND THE FOUNTAIN OF YOUTH

The free radical theory of aging was first proposed by Denham Harman, MD, PhD, a scientist who published his first paper on this theory in 1954. He said free radicals come from water, which is a perfect balance of two hydrogen atoms and one oxygen atom, all sharing their electrons in harmony. When water is split apart unevenly, such as by the heat inside the cell or the power of sunlight, the free radical is the part that does not get its fair share of electrons. Free radicals try to stabilize themselves by stealing electrons from the lipids, or oils, that make up the skin's membranes. That wouldn't be so bad on its own, but then the damaged lipids turn around and snatch electrons from neighboring lipid molecules. Pretty soon a chain reaction of electron robbery is under way, leaving in its wake a string of crippled lipids, like a run in a nylon stocking.

Antioxidants are simply molecules that have an electron to spare. By giving up their spare ones to the free radical, they stop the series of electron thefts called oxidation—hence the name "antioxidants." Some antioxidants readily give up their electrons and are powerful antioxidants, like vitamin E. Others do so only grudgingly, like most plant compounds, and are weak antioxidants. Almost any type of molecule can be at least to some degree an antioxidant.

Dr. Harman thought that free radicals were the inevitable side effect of the chemistry of life. He explained that the energy needed to power living things produces free radicals, much as sparks are thrown off from the engine of a speeding locomotive. The damage from one spark may be small, but the constant accumulation of damage during a lifetime compromises cell function and eventually causes cells to die off.

Early experiments supported the free radical theory by showing that mice that were fed antioxidants had an increased chance to live to an old age. Notice that they didn't live *longer,* but more of them actually reached the maximum life span.

Dr. Harman's theory was originally pooh-poohed in the medical community, but in the 1980s, when the wider scientific community first learned of the free radical theory of aging, it reacted with unrestrained excitement. Before that, aging seemed inevitable, and any search for a cure was thought to be as fanciful as Ponce de León's wanderings in the Florida marshland. But here was Dr. Harman, declaring with experimental evidence that a specific thing—and one that could be easily measured—was really the cause of human mortality.

And at the time he proposed his theory, the world's experts in free radicals were scientists studying the effects caused by the radiation that had been released from nuclear weapons. Less than ten years after the United States unleashed the atomic bomb on Japan, Dr. Harman was proposing that these same scientists might turn their studies to the age-old quest for eternal life. It was heady stuff—and make no mistake, it still is.

THE CHALLENGE FOR ANTIOXIDANTS

Further research showed that there are many types of free radicals, and not every antioxidant can stop every free radical. So right away it is clear that a mixture of antioxidants would seem to be needed in skin if free radical therapy is going to work.

There is an additional complication. In skin, free radicals can be formed in either the water portion or the lipid portion of the cells. The water portion is the soup that composes about 97 percent of the entire cell. But the lipid portion is very important, because lipids form the membranes that separate the cells from one another. Since oil and water don't mix, these really are two completely different environments of life.

Unfortunately, antioxidants are either oil soluble or water soluble, and an oil-soluble antioxidant can't work in the water portion of your skin. You can see immediately that it is impossible for a single type of antioxidant to protect all the parts of the skin from all the types of free radicals.

In your skin, there's an interlaced antioxidant system made up of enzymes and delicate molecules. Skin has one enzyme (superoxide dismutase) to convert singlet oxygen into hydrogen peroxide and two enzymes (catalase and peroxidase), whose job it is to convert hydrogen peroxide and other free radicals into water. Skin is also loaded with four chemical antioxidants. Three of them (ergothioneine, glutathione, and vitamin C) are found in the water portion of skin, and the other (vitamin E) is found in the oil and membrane portions.

ANTIOXIDANTS IN FOODS AND SUPPLEMENTS

So where do we go looking for good antioxidants? Let's start with the foods we eat. Since we consume huge quantities of plant antioxidants in a typical diet, it's worth taking a look at whether this is any good for you or not. Then we'll focus on whether such a diet is any good for your skin in particular.

ANTIOXIDANT FOODS

Without a doubt, the consumption of foods containing antioxidants is good for your body. It lowers the risk of cancer and heart disease. The most convincing evidence came from studies of people who ate whole foods containing a mixture of antioxidants. One study of the eating habits of more than 80,000 nurses found that those who ate foods rich in antioxidants, particularly spinach and carrots, had significantly lower rates of arteriosclerosis and stroke. Adding just three vegetable servings a day reduced the risk of stroke by 22 percent, and a diet with fruit and vegetables at each meal reduced the risk for many types of cancer by half.

The National Academy of Sciences recognizes that there's something special about the mixture of antioxidants found in food and emphasizes that foods—rather than nutritional supplements—are the preferred source of antioxidants.

Foods with Antioxidant Benefits

Broccoli

Cabbage

Carrots

Cauliflower

Citrus fruits

Egg yolks

Garlic

Green tea

Onion

Peppers

Pumpkin

Red grapes

Spinach

Strawberry

Sunflower seeds

Sweet potato

ANTIOXIDANT SUPPLEMENTS

Antioxidant supplements are the nutrients purified from food and put into pills. There have been many studies over many years on what antioxidant supplements do or do not do for the skin, and the evidence so far has been overwhelming. And it's not what you want to hear! So far, it has not been proven that antioxidant supplements have an effect on skin aging, or for that matter that they can reduce your skin cancer risk.

Several studies involving thousands of people who consumed enough beta-carotene from carrots to turn their skin orange did not show any reduction in skin cancer risk. Dr. Homer Black, professor of dermatology at Houston's Baylor College of Medicine and a world expert on the effect of diet on skin, recently warned that not only does beta-carotene not protect against cancer, but in combination with some foods it might actually increase the cancer risk.[1]

The truth is that while foods contain an undefined mixture of both recognized and unknown antioxidants, antioxidant supplements are designed to give you only specific recognized antioxidants in a pill, in amounts far greater than what could possibly be consumed in a balanced diet. As the National Academy of Sciences notes, the evidence that these antioxidant supplements provide any health benefit is much shakier than the nutritional supplement industry lets on. Once in a while, you might read an article reporting that an antioxidant supplement did perform well in a clinical study, but just wait—the next week a story with the opposite conclusion will fill the headlines.

To help end this confusion, in 2004 the Center for Clinical Intervention Research in Copenhagen published their analysis of fourteen human clinical trials that included 170,525 participants. The volunteers in all these studies had taken antioxidant supplements containing beta-carotene, vitamin A, vitamin C, and vitamin E. The conclusion? "We could not find evidence that antioxidant supplements prevent gastrointestinal cancers. On the contrary, they seem to increase overall mortality."[2] The researchers then went on to analyze a total of sixty-eight studies with more than 230,000 participants. Their conclusions, published in 2007, were the same.[3]

This is alarming because too much of an antioxidant can actually turn it into a pro-oxidant—a chemical that *generates* free radicals— which is what you were trying to prevent in the first place! Another study published in 2005 by British scientists showed that a 500-mg megadose of vitamin C actually increases DNA damage.

There is no point in taking megadoses of vitamins C and E in supplement form, because the body regulates their levels and excretes the excess in your urine. Vitamin A, however, is a different story, as it's stored in the body. Too much beta-carotene, which the body converts into vitamin A, increases the risk of heart disease. For smokers, it increases their risk of lung cancer (as if smoking weren't bad enough!).

There are always those who will say that the studies on antioxidants didn't last long enough or the antioxidant doses weren't high enough, and maybe that is true. A new research strategy is also looking for the best combinations of antioxidants that might actually work together synergistically. But in the meantime, millions of people consume fistfuls of supplement tablets daily in the hope that they may have hit upon the right mix. In moderation, it probably doesn't hurt to have a few antioxidants in a daily vitamin supplement, and many vitamins have other benefits in the skin beyond their antioxidant properties.

The real goal of vitamin therapy should be to try to get the optimum mixture through food instead of pills, so the vitamins will have their natural bioprogramming effect. The recommended daily allowance (RDA) on a bottle of vitamins spells this out clearly. And because vitamins have many other functions in the body, their use when it comes to anti-aging might have nothing whatsoever to do with free radicals.

Bottom line: If you want to add antioxidants to your diet, eat lots of fruit and vegetables, just like your mom told you to! But there is very little proof that taking antioxidant supplements does your skin any good. Many clinical studies have shown repeatedly that they have little or no effect on aging or skin cancer prevention and that megadoses may actually be harmful!

ANTIOXIDANTS IN SKIN-CARE PRODUCTS

Since gulping down an antioxidant pill doesn't seem to work, what about loading antioxidants directly onto the skin with creams and lotions? This would seem to make a lot of sense, as they should be able to get right to the target, with no delay.

So do they actually work?

Without doubt, many studies in laboratory mice under careful conditions show that skin-care products chock-full of a variety of antioxidants protect mouse skin from the harmful effects of UV lamps. Among the antioxidants that have performed with stellar success in mice are vitamins A, C, and E, as well as beta-carotene, and the mineral selenium. But none of these have had the same success in serious clinical studies where they were applied to people who went out in the sun.

On balance, studies do not show that antioxidants protect human skin from the sun. The skin-care companies use the same tests for antioxidants as they do for moisturizers, and they get the same results as moisturizers without any antioxidants! And almost all the antioxidant testing is done by adding one antioxidant in huge excess, which as we

will see is absolutely the wrong way to use antioxidants. When dermatologists and scientists get together to discuss antioxidants, they agree
that the theory has merit but after all these years the evidence for benefits of application to human skin is sorely lacking.

Since this is a very controversial point, I want to be absolutely clear
about what I believe to be the truth about antioxidants in the skin.

▪ The skin has a few very special, natural antioxidants, some of
which are also vitamins. They work together in teams, not as lone
rangers. Good health means they are maintained by the body at optimum amounts in relation to one another.

▪ Adding an excess of any one antioxidant, or substituting unnatu-
ral ones from plants, doesn't really produce the benefits companies
claim.

▪ Most of the damage caused by the sun is not from free radicals.
As we saw in chapter 6, most damage is caused by sunlight directly absorbed by DNA—without any free radical involved. Therefore, adding
more antioxidants doesn't improve protection against the sun by very
much.

▪ Antioxidants are overrated by all the marketing hype in beauty
and dermatology advertising. That is not to say that they are worthless
or always harmful—only that we should not depend on them to solve all
of our aging problems. The best advice: Keep a healthy balance of the
natural antioxidants in your skin but don't expect them alone to produce
dramatic anti-aging benefits.

Let's take a closer look at some of the touted antioxidants in skin-
care products and at what—if anything—they really deliver.

GREEN TEA

Take green tea. Cosmetics counters are filled with products containing
green tea, or the antioxidant it contains, namely the polyphenol ECGC.[4]
They're usually accompanied by claims that green tea will reduce the effect of photoaging and restore the skin to glorious youth.

The tea plant is cultivated in more than thirty countries around the world, but only 20 percent of its leaves produce green tea. (The remainder is mostly black tea, along with some oolong.) A special processing of green tea keeps the ECGC inside the leaves; it is then released when the leaves are soaked in hot water.

More than eighty studies in mice and other animals published over the last ten years have shown that tea *does* protect against disease. Most of these studies were performed on green tea, and many specifically studied the effects of green tea applied to skin. This research spurred tremendous hope in the scientific community that ECGC could make a real difference in improving the quality and health of people's skin.

However—and this is a *big* however—studies of humans who applied green tea to their skin had mixed results and were generally disappointing. For every small study that shows a benefit in protecting against sunburn, there is another just as rigorous that failed to find any effect. Unfortunately, reports from those negative studies presented at scientific meetings are usually not carried in beauty magazines or newspaper stories! Believe me, all of us who've looked at these results wish it weren't so. But so far, the evidence showing green tea having any appreciable effect on wrinkles or skin cancer in humans is weak. These are not the results that would be expected after the mice responded so well.

Bottom line: Green tea works well on mouse skin, but it hasn't yet been proven to have notable benefits on human skin.

VITAMINS A, C, AND E

Vitamins do many good things in the body that have nothing to do with fighting free radicals. So let's begin by saying that vitamins in skin-care products have benefits whether or not adding them actually helps the antioxidant system. This means, however, that you will lose overall benefits by substituting other antioxidants for these vitamins.

Let's return to that coordinated system of antioxidant enzymes and chemicals inside the skin. These natural antioxidants perform as a finely tuned orchestra, so using skin-care products to maintain these natural levels makes sense. But adding megadoses of antioxidants to an already fragile mix, through either oral supplements or skin-care products, might not be the best idea. Just as adding another string section to an orchestra doesn't make it sound better—in fact, it can sound a lot worse.

Vitamin C is a proven stimulant for the production of collagen. In many ways only now being discovered by molecular biology, it turns on genes that bolster the skin's supporting lining. Yet only a relatively modest amount of vitamin C is needed to do this, and applying it in megadoses will not help; just as with oral supplements, the body will excrete the excess.

Vitamin A programs each layer of the skin to function at its best— it accelerates the genetic program so that cells robustly perform their designated function. This especially means making more collagen to support the skin and puffing up the cells at the basement layer of skin, all resulting in vibrant skin with a gloss on top. The active form of vitamin A is called retinoic acid. Using vitamin A in the form of retinol found in skin cream is a bit of a step down in potency; it must be metabolized into retinoic acid by cells, and this means much of the vitamin A/retinol gets lost during the transformation. Furthermore, skin cells carefully regulate how much retinoic acid is made, so applying excessive amounts of vitamin A/retinol can't force the skin to make more retinoic acid than it is willing to make. Retinol can keep the skin at its optimum but can't push it into overdrive the way retinoic acid can. This is a safety valve for cosmetic products with retinol, where too much is not more effective than the right amount.

Vitamin E is stored in skin cell membranes and makes them smooth and supple. But there is only so much that can be taken up into membranes before they become saturated. As with the other vitamins, an excess of vitamin E just goes to waste.

Bottom line: Vitamins A, C, and E work in an orchestrated way in the skin, aside from any antioxidant activities. Maintaining the naturally optimum levels by using skin-care products containing them has real benefits. However, adding too much, or substituting other antioxidants, makes no sense.

OVERHYPED ANTIOXIDANT INGREDIENTS

Since antioxidants aren't quite as effective when overused as many cosmetic companies advertise and as the beauty media lead us to believe, you need to approach many of the overhyped antioxidant ingredients with a healthy dose of skepticism.

Remember that while an antioxidant can detoxify a free radical, it can also convert one free radical into another. Don't fall for the hype swearing that if an ingredient is an antioxidant, then more of it means more protection from free radicals. The body doesn't work that way. Having too many of the wrong kind of antioxidants skews the reaction and may end up causing more harm than good to your skin. Here are a few problems and pretenders to watch out for on product labels.

"DUSTING"

As we discussed, some companies "dust" a product, which means they sprinkle an almost negligible amount of an active antioxidant ingredient into the product and then proceed to claim all of its supposed benefits. This is really a double whammy for consumers, who are being sold on the "proven" benefits of an antioxidant that isn't even in the product in any measurable quantity! Beware of products when the highly touted "hero" antioxidant appears far down on the ingredient list.

ALPHA-LIPOIC ACID

Alpha-lipoic acid is a much heralded "new antioxidant" and a key ingredient in the N.V. Perricone skin-care line, among many others. Here, the claims are particularly curious, because alpha-lipoic acid is never found alone in the body but always bound to a partner enzyme that actually does all the work (which, by the way, has nothing to do with neutralizing free radicals). So, frankly, adding more alpha-lipoic acid to a skin-care product, without its heavy-lifting partner, should not be expected to produce any effects on its own.

To be fair, a study conducted at the Karolinska University Hospital in Stockholm applied a 5-percent alpha-lipoic acid preparation twice daily for twelve weeks to one half of the faces of thirty-three women and a control cream on the other side of their faces.[5] After this rigorous regimen, the dermatologists did find a 50 percent reduction in "skin roughness" on the alpha-lipoic acid side of the face—but they also found a 40 percent improvement on the placebo side!

Bottom line: The science behind alpha-lipoic acid doesn't make much sense. As I've already discussed, the placebo effect can be very potent, and the use of *any* moisturizer, with our without alpha-lipoic acid, will improve skin texture.

IDEBENONE

Allergan Dermatology's answer to CoQ10 was to introduce idebenone, a lab-made, oil-soluble antioxidant with a similar chemical structure. Idebenone at 1 percent strength was initially sold as Prevage MD, and it was available only at doctors' offices. Elizabeth Arden subsequently introduced a Prevage serum containing 0.5 percent idebenone into retail stores. Allergan claims that idebenone is the strongest antioxidant known to man, but recently published research from our lab shows that ergothioneine is even stronger!

Idebenone was heavily promoted as being able to reverse all the signs of aging, including wrinkles, uneven skin tone, and sagging. In one full-page ad in *The New York Times,* Dr. Kenneth Hertz of Miami was quoted under "Proof Not Promises" as saying, "Prevage is clinically proven to protect the skin." But when I wrote to Dr. Hertz to ask about the proof, he replied that he had not done any work in this area personally and that he had simply been asked by Elizabeth Arden to review the studies. So I did that too.

The first paper[6] published on idebenone is an example of how a science experiment can get turned around in an attempt to prove a point. The study looked at five volunteers who agreed to apply idebenone solution to sites on their skin and to have those sites exposed to UV light. The next day, sections of skin were biopsied from each site and then studied under a microscope. What the researchers were looking for were "sunburn cells," which are easily recognized by their dark, knotty appearance. They didn't find as many of these cells in the idebenone-treated skin, so they concluded that the treated skin had been protected.

At Yale University, Dr. David Leffell, a dermatology professor, and Dr. Douglas Brash, a professor of therapeutic radiology, have been studying sunburn cells in skin together for more than a decade. They concluded that a sunburn cell is the waste by-product of skin repair—not unlike trash from a construction site that is put out for collection in a Dumpster. What Leffell and Brash have found, however, is that skin that has *failed* to repair damage, and therefore does not produce any "trash," also has fewer sunburn cells.

So what does this mean? The absence of sunburn cells can mean either that damage was prevented or that there was no repair. So we can't really say from the published study cited above, as the Prevage advertising asserts, that the idebenone is providing any benefit proven by sunburn cells. It certainly has nothing to do with wrinkles.

Another idebenone study used forty-one women, who applied either 1 percent or 0.5 percent idebenone for six weeks. There was no placebo or any other product to compare it against, and the subjects had to stop using any other anti-aging product in order to be in the study. Not surprisingly under these conditions, the subjects' skin became more hydrated, with fewer wrinkles, over the six weeks—which only proves that something (almost anything) is better than nothing. What was surprising was that there was almost no difference in results between the 1 percent and 0.5 percent idebenone formulas—especially so because the 1 percent formula is sold only in doctors' offices as medical grade and the 0.5 percent formula is sold in stores as the more mild form! In this study it seems the moisturizing and antiwrinkle effect took place regardless of the amount of idebenone—or maybe without it at all?

Bottom line: Idebenone may be a strong antioxidant, but it can't do the job by itself. In Prevage, it's going solo in the antiwrinkle fight, armed only with a moisturizing effect. The proof that it works is just not there.

THE ANTIOXIDANTS THAT REALLY WORK

Instead of falling for the typical antioxidant hype, let's take a look at what the properly balanced antioxidant products of the New Skin-Care Revolution *can* do. These products focus on placing antioxidants directly where they can really deliver benefits—by using them *in teams* to optimize the natural antioxidants of the skin, keeping up the level of vitamins, and by protecting DNA. The goal here is to keep the optimum natural healthy level of antioxidants, which can become depleted by poor skin care, too much sun and pollution, and too much exfoliation.

Antioxidants and Exfoliating Treatments

Exfoliation is more popular than ever, whether in the form of at-home peel kits; OTC microdermabrasion creams; alpha-hydroxy acid; beta- and polyhydroxy acid chemical peels; or deeper microdermabrasion and laser treatments at the dermatologist's office.

Without question, exfoliation produces immediate benefits. Your skin will be clearer, with a more even tone. Many of the signs of accumulated photoaging, such as fine lines, hyperpigmentation, and sallowness, will be diminished. Why, your skin might even seem to have a glow to it.

All this is to say that the right amount of exfoliation is good for your skin. But—and this is a big but—exfoliation works so well because it strips away part of the stratum corneum, your skin's topmost layer. Too much of that is never good.

The problem with exfoliation is that much of the skin's antioxidants and vitamins, particularly vitamins C and E, are embedded in the stratum corneum. Stripping them away means your skin is essentially robbed of some of its supplies. As a result, your skin will be out of balance until it can be naturally replenished. The more you peel, in fact, the less time you give your skin to rebuild its defenses.

THE ADVANTAGES OF TEAMS

We've learned that an antioxidant molecule must be at the right place at the right time to intercept the free radical before it does its damage. Remember, free radicals show up in both the water and oil portions of the skin, but a single antioxidant can't go after both areas. For example, vitamin C can only patrol the water zone, while CoQ10 is insoluble in water and only works in the lipid zone. So, for antioxidant preparations to be truly effective, they have to contain both water soluble *and* oil soluble ingredients. This way, they can capture singlet oxygen and also smother hydroxyl radicals while protecting DNA from damage.

Another reason that it's better for antioxidants to team up is that they get tired! Reacting with free radicals often exhausts them, and they can only be regenerated by other antioxidants operating as medics.

Exfoliation is one of the most common examples of an unintended consequence—a skin rejuvenation technique that does one good thing (tackling the effects of photoaging) while creating a potentially bad thing (destroying skin's natural healthy balance of antioxidants and vitamins).

Bottom line: If you are happy with your exfoliating treatments, feel free to stick with them. But at the same time, you should do your utmost to restore the lost antioxidants and vitamins you have deliberately stripped away. This can easily be done by following any exfoliation treatment with a carefully formulated antioxidant cream. It should contain vitamins A, C, and E, and it should have a moisturizing base. Be sure to use this type of cream after any procedure that disrupts or removes the stratum corneum.

For much more information about exfoliation, see chapter 10.

Postexfoliation Antioxidant Creams

* Cellex-C Advanced-C Serum
* Remergent Antioxidant Refoliator
  Post-Peel Balm
* SkinCeuticals C E Ferulic
* Skin Culture Matrix Booster

When, for instance, vitamin E becomes exhausted after stopping chain reactions in the cell's membranes, vitamin C steps in to recycle the spent vitamin E and restore the antioxidant capacity of these membranes. And when vitamin C is worn out, it is also then recycled by other antioxidants in the cell. When that happens, the whole sequence is set back into motion. In essence, the natural antioxidant system is a harmonious and continual recycling of radical-busting players.

Since it is impossible for a solo antioxidant ingredient to work effectively on all free radicals, you can discard all the hype by those products promoting their "wonder" solo-hero ingredients. What you need is a product that has carefully combined a mixture of different antioxidants that can reach all the parts of the cells in your skin and then are able to recycle one another and maintain their protective effect.

Bottom line: For products to be effective, they need to be formulated with integrated antioxidants so that they can reach all parts of the cells and then recycle one another when they are exhausted.

THE WINNING TEAMS

The best candidates for teamed-up antioxidants are the major natural vitamins found in the skin—vitamins C and E and ergothioneine. On their own the vitamins are too unstable to be consistently effective in skin-care products. Most have lost their potency before you've even brought them home from the store! Luckily, there is a way around this problem. Vitamins can be modified by adding on a chemical tag—a short string of harmless molecules that stabilize them like the tail of a kite in the wind. This chemical tag can also improve absorption into the skin; once the tag enters, it is cut off inside the cell and the pure vitamin remains. Tagged forms of vitamins C and E are less efficiently used in cells because of this extra cleavage step, but they certainly are a start—especially when mixed together in the right combination.

RECOMMENDED VITAMIN TEAMS OF ANTIOXIDANTS

- ❋ Cellex-C Advanced-C Serum
- ❋ Cosmedicine MegaDose Skin Fortifying Serum
- ❋ H_2O Plus Face Oasis Hydrating Treatment
- ❋ MDSkincare Anti-Aging Vitamin C Gel
- • Olay Total Effects 7X Visible Anti-Aging Vitamin Complex with UV Protection
- ❋ Remergent Antioxidant Refoliator Post-Peel Balm (with ergothioneine)
- ❋ SkinCeuticals C E Ferulic

HOW AND WHEN TO USE ANTIOXIDANTS

As you grow older, the amount of antioxidants stored in your skin begins to decline. If you start using a potent antioxidant in your twenties or thirties, you will give yourself a lifetime of optimal antioxidant levels.

But if you're older than that, don't despair. It's not too late to reverse the effects of aging, and you can start to do this by restoring youthful levels of antioxidants.

The goal here is not to overwhelm the skin with a ridiculous amount of one particular antioxidant, but to maintain the optimal mixture of vitamins and antioxidants at all times. This is particularly important as sun exposure not only decimates the antioxidants in your skin, but creates a vicious cycle where the degraded molecules create more free radicals. Surprisingly few sunscreen makers recognize this fact.

Here are a few more tips:

▪ Don't rely exclusively on antioxidant products to reduce wrinkles, because free radicals are not the only, and maybe not even the most important, cause of wrinkles.

▪ For true replenishment and rejuvenation, seek out formulas such as those recommended here that contain stable antioxidants mixed in specific combinations that protect both the water and lipid portions of your skin. The formulation will contain both water-soluble and oil-soluble antioxidants.

▪ Vitamins C and E are important for skin health. Don't substitute other antioxidants for these vitamins in your skin-care products, but be sure the vitamins are stabilized and in combination. Otherwise you'll be wasting your money.

▪ Use good antioxidant products daily to maintain an optimal level in your skin and to repair your DNA. This is especially crucial if you are planning to spend extra time in the sun, such as on a vacation, or after any exfoliation treatment, no matter how mild.

Although I already mentioned these sunscreens in chapter 6, they are worth repeating here.

RECOMMENDED SUNSCREENS WITH ANTIOXIDANTS

- Lancôme Bienfait Multi-Vital SPF 30 Sunscreen
- ☀ Murasun Daily Sunblock with Antioxidants SPF 15

- ☀ Pharmaskincare Cover Mild SPF 15 Antioxidant
- ☀ Remergent A.M. Moisture SPF 15 Sunscreen
- ☀ Remergent High Intensity SPF 30 Sunscreen

DNA REPAIR ANTIOXIDANTS

The first truly new antioxidants in decades are finally here. These antioxidants repair damaged DNA. And they work!

One of the most typical reactions in a cell is when DNA is damaged when a free radical attaches itself to the DNA molecule. It's so typical, in fact, that nearly every living thing has a special repair enzyme whose sole function is to fix this damage. This DNA repair enzyme is called OGG1.

Our laboratory at AGI Dermatics has taken the OGG1 enzyme found in the tiny *Arabidopsis* mustard plant and packed it in liposomes that deliver it precisely into skin cells. Once there, this special enzyme carries a signal that sends it to the two places inside a cell where DNA is found: the nucleus and the mitochondria. Testing has shown that it then specifically helps speed removal of the oxidized DNA in both locations.

This is a very real scientific breakthrough. Mitochondria are especially important to skin because they are the powerhouses of the cell and produce the energy that allows cells to divide and grow. Damage to mitochondrial DNA has been linked to premature aging. Being able to repair DNA there means that skin can work at full throttle, which brings that rosy, healthy glow. It's not too late to repair DNA, especially mitochondrial DNA, at any age and recover the optimum vitality of skin.

Bottom line: Today, even free radical damage to DNA can be fixed. New products are able to enhance and optimize the normal repair, especially protecting the skin's energy production.

RECOMMENDED DNA REPAIR ANTIOXIDANTS

- ☀ Esteé Lauder Re-Nutriv Ultimate Lifting Serum
- ☀ Remergent Antioxidant Refoliator Post-Peel Balm
- ☀ Remergent DNA Repair Formula

THE NEWEST NATURAL ANTIOXIDANT:
ERGOTHIONEINE

As I wrote in chapter 5, ergothioneine is one of the new generations of antioxidants that is a natural amino acid. It is found at high concentrations both in the human bloodstream, where it protects hemoglobin from oxidation, and in the eye, where it protects the lenses from cataracts. Our laboratory has recently discovered that it is a natural component of our skin's defense system. Our bodies don't make ergothioneine, so we need to get it from food, most notably grains and vegetables.

A remarkably stable antioxidant, ergothioneine can withstand near-boiling temperatures for several days without breaking down. In addition, it's recycled in cells when partnered with vitamin C. In published research spanning eighty years, ergothioneine has been shown to be a powerful antioxidant, eliminating both singlet oxygen and hydroxyl radicals. Plus, it assists cells in the process of making more energy while soaking up any excess free radicals that might be created in the process. It also helps clarify skin and reduce hyperpigmentation. Best of all, in head-to-head antioxidant tests, ergothioneine outperforms vitamins C and E and both CoQ10 and idebenone.

Bottom line: If you want to be in the forefront of the New Skin-Care Revolution, ergothioneine is one of the best skin-care ingredients you can use. Nevertheless, it still should be formulated with a team of antioxidants, as it is in the following products.

RECOMMENDED ERGOTHIONEINE ANTIOXIDANT PRODUCTS

* Botáge IDB Facial Anti-oxidant Formula
* Cellex-C Advanced-C Serum
* Dior No Age Essentiel Progress Age-Defying Refining Cream
* Elizabeth Arden Ceramide Eye Wish
* Kinerase Hydrating Antioxidant Mist
* Kinerase Lip Treatment
* Neways Rebound

Pros and Cons of
Isoflavones/Plant Estrogens

The trend toward identifying and extracting antioxidants from botanicals has uncovered some interesting new antioxidants, particularly isoflavones. These are also known as plant estrogens, or phytoestrogens, since they can bind to estrogen receptors on human cells and mimic the effects of the female hormone estrogen. The best known and studied is genistein, which comes from soybeans.

In the laboratory, purified isoflavones show antioxidant activity at concentrations that are usually higher than those found in cosmetics containing other flowers, plant extracts, or soy protein. One team at the University of Michigan found that pure genistein applied to the skin of human volunteers blocked many of the effects of the sun's damaging UV rays. This is a very promising result, and it may have nothing to do with isoflavones being antioxidants, but rather because they act like hormones.

Be careful when choosing a soy product, though, especially if you have a family history of breast cancer or any hormonal imbalance. On the one hand, estrogen supplements relieve the symptoms of perimenopause and menopause when natural estrogen levels begin to fall. On the other hand, estrogens increase the risk of breast cancer, especially those cancers with receptors that feed off estrogen. If a phytoestrogen like genistein is to work at all on your skin, it may stimulate estrogen receptors—and this suggests a cancer risk. In addition, several cases have been reported of young men who developed marked breast enlargement from using shampoos containing lavender and tea tree oils, essential oils full of phytoestrogens and widely found in cosmetics. Pregnant women

* Neways Retention Plus
* Neways Skin Enhancer
* Remergent Barrier Repair Formula
* Remergent Clarifying Concentrate[2]
* Zenyaku Kogyo Gelée Rich Pure Injuvenate Essence

should not add flaxseed oil to their diet or their skin. The consumption of flaxseed oil, which is high in phytoestrogens, may lead to developmental abnormalities in the fetus.

As yet, there's not been a good clinical study that has shown an increase in cancer risk from any soy product or from soy consumption. Many skin-care formulas use soy protein (without the isoflavones and phytoestrogens) that can't claim the benefits of isoflavones but probably are not a health risk.

Always discuss the use of any skin-care product featuring high concentrations of soy isoflavones or other phytoestrogens with your doctor, especially as you approach menopause. You certainly should not risk your health because you want to get rid of wrinkles!

Bottom line: The benefits of isoflavones are encouraging, but they carry some potential risk. They are best suited to younger women who are not pregnant.

RECOMMENDED MOISTURIZERS WITH ISOFLAVONES AND PLANT ESTROGENS

- Aveeno Positively Radiant Daily Moisturizer SPF 15
- DDF Silky C (with retinol, soy, and lutein)
- Earth Therapeutics Clari-T First Aid Kit
- KaplanMD Phytogenic Triactive Complex Perfecting Serum
- Lamas Botanicals Soy Nourishing Moisturizer
- Reviva Labs Soy Intensive Rejuvenating Serum
- SoySoft Daily Moisturizing Body Lotion

■   ■   ■

Wrinkle Treatments

Nowhere is the noise and confusion of competing product claims more deafening than in the quest to get rid of wrinkles.

For those of us working in the New Skin-Care Revolution, it's incredibly ironic. Right now, brand-new skin-renewing solutions that really work are bursting out of laboratories. At the same time, many cosmetic companies are making outrageous and entirely ridiculous claims about products that don't live up to the hype. Not that long ago, cosmetics ads first claimed to be able to reduce wrinkles in one month . . . then one week . . . then one day . . . and then overnight. Overnight? That's way too long! Why, a recent ad for Lancôme's Primordiale Optimum line featured a stopwatch, promising wrinkle removal in *five seconds*. The ultimate promise, of course, was made by Dr. Nicholas Perricone. In the title of his first book, published in 2000, he announced to the world that he had a wrinkle "cure"—a term not used lightly in the medical community.

So consumers try these products, don't see anywhere near that kind of improvement, feel cheated or enraged by all the bombastic baloney, and then give up. They don't know that help really is there—if you keep your expectations realistic and you know where to look for it. Those who are in step with the New Skin-Care Revolution know that there are amazing products that target deeper wrinkles, the kind of damage in the lower levels of your skin that has accumulated over decades of sun exposure. And you'll get even better results when partnering these new creams with the retinoids, AHAs, and collagen-remodeling peels that have already been proven to work on fine lines.

ABOUT WRINKLES

Wrinkles are more complex than most of us realize.

If you peer through a microscope at a cross section of wrinkled skin, the changes are easily visible. In some areas, the surface skin will be noticeably dry, with creases and cracks. This is where the cells on the surface have produced fewer ceramides. In the lower level, the dermis, the supporting fabric of collagen and elastin has diminished, having been digested by an ever-rising level of corrosive enzymes. This leads to a loss of elasticity. Add the inescapable fact that skin normally loses volume as we age, since the fat that plumps up younger skin is gradually reabsorbed by your body over the years, and we can only reach one conclusion: Minimizing wrinkles, getting rid of them, and keeping new ones from forming is a very tricky process.

When you examine wrinkled skin under the higher magnification of an electron microscope, it appears as though the intertwined cables of collagen and elastin proteins supporting the skin have been ruptured. The fibroblast cells that knit the collagen cables together have been pulled apart. Wherever the torn streaks appear—and they're most visible in areas of frequent flexing, like the outer corner of the eyes and around the mouth—the skin has already begun to lose the cushioned packing of fat. As a result, when creases form, they can't snap back.

Bottom line: Many wrinkles are caused by a series of changes in the skin as it ages and are not just a simple one-step problem to be fixed. Welcome to the aging process. Believe it or not, this is all a normal part of intrinsic aging. It happens to everyone, although each body is, of course, slightly different, following its unique genetic program.

PHOTOAGING

The sun triggers similar responses in skin, but when you examine sun-damaged skin under the electron microscope, photoaging tells an entirely different story. The skin's topmost layer has thickened in defense, not unlike the calluses that form on your heels and toes. Deeper down, the collagen and elastin bundles that give the skin its bouncy strength are no longer recognizable. Not only are the collagen bundles punctured, but in many places they've been so completely digested that none remain at all. Instead, fragments of individual fibers are strewn about, and the spaces are filled with collagen debris. The fibroblast cells of the lower layer are not just separated but are no longer attached to intact collagen. They lie isolated, surrounded by wreckage.

A common misperception is that sunlight beaming directly into your skin destroys the collagen layer by letting loose free radicals, which then create this wasteland of fragments and rubble. What really happens is that sunlight wounds the upper layer of living cells, and in response they release an enzyme, called matrix metalloproteinase 1 (MMP-1). This enzyme literally chews down collagen and elastin fiber bundles from one end to the other, leaving a mess behind.

If you scrape your skin, two other MMPs, called MMP-2 and MMP-9 (the good guys), jump to action, like the cleanup crew after a hurricane. They sanitize the degraded collagen fibers by quickly reducing them to pulp, which is swept away via microcirculation. Even though some of the collagen is gone, the remaining fibroblast cells remain anchored to residual full-length collagen cables.

Not so in photoaged skin. MMP-1 released by injured cells is working overtime to chew up collagen. At the same time, however, the MMP-2 and MMP-9 cleanup crews fail to arrive—they are missing in action! As a result, chopped-up collagen trash is strewn about the lower level of skin, and this prevents new collagen from forming.

This miniature war zone, called a microscar, is the result of a single bout with the sun. Multiplied over decades, these microscars coalesce.

And you end up with a face full of wrinkles.

Bottom line: Wrinkles caused by sunlight are entirely different from intrinsic aging wrinkles, and they require a completely different strategy to make use of the body's own natural healing process.

VITAMIN POWER

The most powerful forces in the war against wrinkles have been two vitamins, A and C.

Vitamins are organic molecules that serve primarily to stimulate metabolism in the body. If they are in short supply, normal body functions break down. Getting the RDA for vitamins is essential for good health and is easy enough to do if you eat a balanced diet and/or take a good daily supplement.

But getting vitamins, famous for their instability outside of food, to function in skin-care products has been a problem from day one. Luckily, there are enough top-quality products available so that you can harness vitamins' power to combat wrinkles.

THE POWER OF VITAMIN A: RETINOIC ACID AND RETINOL
Retinoic Acid
Vitamin A, found mainly in red and green vegetables, is converted by the body from beta-carotene into retinol and then into retinoic acid. For many years it was thought that the main benefit of vitamin A was in sharpening eyesight. Vitamin A's dramatic skin-care benefits were revealed in 1979, in the first wave of the Skin-Care Revolution, by Albert Kligman, MD, PhD, a professor of dermatology at the University of Pennsylvania, who was working on an acne medication. His acne patients in their thirties and forties began to report that not only was retinoic acid keeping their breakouts under control, but they were seeing improvements in their wrinkles, blotchiness, skin tone, and texture. Their photoaged skin was literally being rejuvenated. In 1984, Dr. Kligman and his colleagues announced that topical tretinoin, to be called Retin-A, enhanced the repair of dermal connective tissue damaged by sunlight.

Retinoic acid has the remarkable ability to reprogram skin cells into behaving as if they were baby cells sprung fresh from the dermis. Instead of producing collagen-degrading enzymes, they produce more collagen. As a result, the stratum corneum thins, the lower layer plumps up, and fine lines and brown spots are reduced.

Once approved by the FDA, prescription Retin-A became a huge hit for women of all ages, whether or not they had acne. One drawback to all tretinoin drugs is that they can't alter the gene itself, or its DNA, so you need to keep using them if their anti-aging effects are to last. But no other skin-rejuvenation therapy has been proven better in large-scale double-blind testing to remove fine wrinkling, lighten brown spots and other discolorations, and to smooth out rough skin. With regular use, tretinoin leaves the skin not just with the appearance of youth, but demonstrably clearer, smoother, firmer, and more pliant.

Unfortunately, retinoic acid has very real side effects. As it thins the skin's topmost layer, it makes skin much more easily sunburned, so all retinoic acid and related products come with a special sun warning to use a sunscreen religiously or risk a severe burn. And this thinner skin layer also allows water to escape more easily, leaving skin dry and flaky.

You have to pay attention to your skin if you use retinoic acid. In order to see real results, you have to be prepared for the occasional bout of sun sensitivity, dry skin, and peeling. And there's a fine line between good-bye to fewer wrinkles and an overly dry, irritated condition.

This is no reason not to use retinoic acid. Discuss options with your dermatologist, as retinoic acid comes in different versions, some of which are less drying than others. Those who find Renova (tretinoin with a moisturizer mixed in) too drying might try adapalene, called Differin, which is less irritating but less effective and technically only FDA approved for the treatment of acne. A third and newer alternative is tazarotene, called Avage, which is approved for treating acne and plaque psoriasis.

Bottom line: Retinoic acid is the active form of vitamin A that dramatically changes the way in which the genetic program is expressed in skin, thinning the upper layer and visibly reducing wrinkles. This comes at the cost of dry and sun-sensitive skin.

Retinol

Prescription retinoic acid drugs soon found themselves in competition with their OTC cousin, retinol. As retinol is less expensive and less potent—and therefore less likely to cause irritation—it's an ideal compromise for cosmetics.

Bear in mind that there are good reasons why retinol is a weaker cousin. Vitamin A is extremely sensitive to light and heat and can quickly degrade. (Nature preserves it by binding it to chemical carrier molecules.) Retinol will always be an unstable vitamin, and unless special precautions are taken, any potency will be quickly lost from most skin-care products.

The human body stores ingested vitamin A in its preserved bound form. If the skin's level of retinoic acid falls too low, the stored vitamin A is retrieved and converted into active retinoic acid. So retinol in cosmetics needs to be converted into retinoic acid by the body, too. It's hard to get too much retinoic acid from retinol because the body controls the amount it converts—but as with Retin-A, this means you need to keep using enough retinol to increase natural levels of retinoic acid.

And, of course, you must always protect your skin from the sun if you use any retinol product.

Bottom line: Retinol is a less potent form of vitamin A that still retains some of retinoic acid's benefits and lessens its risks.

RECOMMENDED RETINOL PRODUCTS

- EmerginC Multi-Vitamin and Retinol Serum
- MD Formulations Vit-A-Plus line
- Neutrogena Healthy Skin Anti-Wrinkle Cream
- Replenix Retinol Smoothing Serum 10X
- RoC Retinol Correxion Deep Wrinkle Daily Moisturizer

THE POWER OF VITAMIN C

The other vitamin with proven wrinkle-fighting power is vitamin C, also known as ascorbic acid. Vitamin C works deep within the skin to stimulate collagen production. No other antioxidant can substitute for vitamin C's particular contribution to the war on wrinkles—which is, however, not directly related to vitamin C's antioxidant power.

Vitamin C has several unique properties that increase the skin's stabilizing structure. It switches on the genes that make collagen, stimulates enzymes that keep pumping out collagen and binding them into cables, and it stops enzymes that degrade collagen. Unfortunately, as we age from twenty to fifty, the levels of vitamin C in our skin can drop by 35 percent—leading to more microscars and more wrinkling. So adding it to an anti-aging regimen seems like a good idea.

There are several drawbacks to vitamin C, however. One is that it diminishes the levels of elastin, another type of cable in the skin. This might be a concern, since skin doesn't normally make more elastin after maturity; what you see is what you've got. The long-term effects of vita- · min C on elastin have not been explored in depth. Another drawback is that too much vitamin C can be toxic to cells, so the body carefully regulates its levels. Unneeded vitamin C is excreted in the urine.

Despite the elastin question, vitamin C would be considered a miracle wrinkle cure if it were not for two major problems. The first is that it penetrates very slowly down to the lower layers of skin where collagen is made, even though it's readily absorbed into the stratum corneum. This means you need a large concentration (5, 10, or even 15 percent of the final formula) of vitamin C—it takes hours or even days after application to be able to measure any increase in the dermis. So you should never believe any claim that a vitamin C cream starts to protect your skin instantly!

The second major problem with vitamin C is that its pure form, ascorbic acid, is unstable. It readily dissipates when dissolved in water at room temperature.

Never fear—cosmetic chemists have developed diverse ways of stabilizing vitamin C. The best way is to bind it up with metals in the form of magnesium ascorbyl phosphate (MAP). Other methods are to convert it from its water-soluble form into an oil-soluble storage form, making compounds like ascorbyl palmitate. But these methods come at a price—stabilized vitamin C must be unpacked by skin enzymes from these storage forms in order to activate it. This diminishes its immediate potency, too.

The best suggestion for any vitamin C products is to keep them away from sunlight and use them up quickly. Avoid storing any vitamin C products for more than six to nine months.

Bottom line: Vitamin C is a leader in collagen building and wrinkle fighting, although its long-term effects on the skin's elastin are unknown. High concentrations and several days are needed to see its effects on reprogramming skin. On balance, vitamin C is one of the ingredients that we can say with certainty works to benefit skin.

RECOMMENDED VITAMIN C PRODUCTS

* Cellex-C Advanced-C Serum
* Remergent Antioxidant Refoliator Post-Peel Balm
* SkinCeuticals C E Ferulic

EXFOLIATION AND AHAS/PHAS/BHAS

Alpha-hydroxy acids, also known as AHAs, continued the Skin-Care Revolution when they were first launched in the late 1980s. Far gentler than the strong phenol and trichloroacetic acid peels used by dermatologists to remove fine lines and wrinkles, AHAs are primarily derived from fruit and milk products. They work by speeding up the loss of dead skin cells and thinning the stratum corneum, and in the process they produce a tingling sensation. The key mechanism of AHAs is setting off a wound-healing response in the lower dermis, which triggers increased collage production and has a visible antiwrinkle effect.

The combination of fewer wrinkles (even if they are the fine-line variety), smoother skin, and freshened color can produce a remarkable change in your complexion. Even better, changes usually happen quickly, sometimes in only a few days.

The introduction of AHAs into skin care was a truly groundbreaking change that other products have often struggled to match. What's more, many AHA users have grown to expect a mild tingling sensation, which not only produces a blush on the skin, but signals that these products are *live* and effective. That tingle, however, is hard to distinguish from the mild irritation of a poorly formulated product. Whatever the outcome, though, the AHA tingle has raised expectations of the way treatment products should feel on skin.

The first AHAs were glycolic acid and lactic acid, in concentrations of up to 10 percent; stronger solutions must be given by a dermatologist, as they can burn the skin. OTC concentrations of glycolic and lactic acid can stink and burn, so the search was on for less irritating alternatives.

Many exfoliating products now contain PHAs (polyhydroxy acids, such as gluconolactone and lactobionic acid). PHAs are AHAs that have been chemically modified to be gentler. BHAs (such as salicylic acid) are cousins of AHAs but are more oil soluble. They are also stronger, more irritating, and not as widely used.

Some companies have tried to reduce AHA irritation by increasing the pH (thereby reducing the acidity) of the formulations. But there's still no getting around the fact that AHAs and PHAs work *because* they're acids, and in order for them to exfoliate properly they must be significantly more acidic than normal skin. "Neutralized" AHA skin-care products are, in effect, useless.

Another fairly recent development is home microdermabrasion creams, which contain scrubbing granules. They roughly strip away the top layer of skin but aren't as potent as AHA and PHA creams, which lift off the upper layer by chemical means. You shouldn't use both, as that would be overkill and could cause unnecessary irritation. The scrubbing granules may be good at cleansing, but they don't achieve the reduction in fine lines and wrinkles that AHA products do.

What everyone should understand about exfoliants is that, yes, they are terrific at removing wrinkles and increasing collagen production, but they still have a very real side effect. The stratum corneum may be composed of dead skin cells, but it shouldn't be thought of as a useless shroud trapping the vital, living skin beneath. Far from it, in fact! The stratum corneum is loaded with antioxidants to absorb the toxic effects of pollution and the sun without letting harm come to the skin. A large portion of all the vitamin C, vitamin E, and other antioxidants in the skin is blended into these top layers of skin. The stratum corneum itself also helps to deflect the sun.

It is absolutely crucial to replace these antioxidants after exfoliation. Whenever you are exfoliating, you need a second step that will ensure that you are restoring antioxidant vitamins. And, of course, sunscreen use in the daytime, especially when exfoliating, is an absolute must.

Bottom line: AHAs are in the front line of wrinkle reduction. The newer PHAs avoid some of their harshness. Care must be used because these products do thin the upper layer of skin, strip away antioxidants, and make skin more sensitive to sun.

HOW TO USE AHA AND PHA EXFOLIANTS

AHA and PHA products are best used at night for six to twelve weeks in order to achieve the peeling effect. Apply them after cleansing and let them sink in before covering the skin with moisturizer. Be sure to wash carefully the next morning to help remove the exfoliated skin cells, and follow with an antioxidant replenishing moisturizer.

Stop using them for six weeks to allow for recovery, to reduce sun sensitivity, and to allow the benefits of the wound-healing response to kick in. At low concentrations, AHAs and PHAs increase the effectiveness of certain other active ingredients that do other things, such as skin lightening, by stimulating cell turnover and triggering collagen production. But for pure exfoliation, it's best to use AHA and PHA products on their own, so look for those that have not been combined with other active ingredients.

RECOMMENDED AHA AND PHA EXFOLIANTS

- ✸ GlyDerm Cream Plus 10% (10 percent glycolic acid)
- ✸ M.D. Forté Lotion I (15 percent glycolic acid)
- ✸ NeoStrata Exuviance Rejuvenating Complex (12 percent polyhydroxy acids)

RECOMMENDED POSTEXFOLIATION ANTIOXIDANTS

- ✸ Cellex-C Advanced-C Serum
- ✸ Remergent Antioxidant Refoliator Post-Peel Balm
- ✸ SkinCeuticals C E Ferulic

DON'T BELIEVE ALL THE
ANTIWRINKLE PROMISES

The wrinkle-busting market is big business—and because it's capitalizing on the hopes and fears of women growing older, it has become a confusing hodgepodge of products with ingredients that work, laced with those that aren't much more than hype and false promises. A lot more research is needed to support some of the candidates. Others just don't make sense altogether!

Let's take a look at the contenders and the pretenders, starting with the ever-popular peptides.

THE BASICS OF PEPTIDES

Peptides are fragments of digested proteins, made up of short chains of amino acids. They don't do any work in the skin. Rather, they are supposed to trigger anti-aging responses by giving the right signals to cells. They are the main claim to fame for a myriad of products, including pricey ones from StriVectin, Perricone, and TNS and drugstore brand names Neutrogena and Olay.

For a scientist it's hard to believe that a small piece of protein could do as much as the whole thing—or else why would we have the whole protein in the first place? The peptide promoters never explain exactly what these peptides are "turning on" in the skin and how digested fragments can be so specific and not turn on anything bad. Think of it this way: if the protein were a phone number, with area code, exchange, and four-digit number, then the peptide would be just the last four digits. The whole protein will ring the right phone in the right city, but the peptide might unnecessarily ring hundreds or thousands of phones across the country, giving you very little chance of talking to the person you want to reach.

A bigger problem with peptides is that an entire piece of protein, or even just a piece of it, can have trouble getting into the skin. The first barrier is that the skin is loaded with enzymes that love to chew on naked proteins and peptides. These enzymes defend us against bacteria and viruses by cutting off their protein attachment probes before they can take hold. This is a good thing—we need this basic defense against proteins entering the skin or else we'd be at the mercy of every surface bacteria and virus that came along. These enzymes aren't picky; to them a protein is a protein, whether it comes in a skin-care peptide or strep or *E. coli.*

Then there are the problems with the size and the electrical charge on peptide molecules. Skin has its own electrical charge on its membranes, again designed to repel bacteria and viruses. So without a sophisticated delivery vehicle to bypass these peptide chompers, you're wasting your time. But if you put a coating on the peptide to protect it, it can't do its job in signaling.

Diabetics know this because insulin is a peptide. If they could rub it into their skin so it would get inside the body, they wouldn't have to inject it with needles every day. But they still use the needles, which should tell you something about whether topical peptides can really work for you.

Despite all this, some products with huge proteins claim to do wonders for wrinkles. DermaLastyl-ß from DermaPlus contains the protein tropoelastin, which makes up elastin, the elastic fibers in the skin that give it stretchiness and bounce. But tropoelastin is 100 times larger than a typical peptide! Hydroderm Age-Defying Fast Acting Wrinkle Reducer says it delivers collagen peptides and even whole collagen into skin. Even if this could happen, it's more likely that the collagen pieces would trigger collagen destruction—just like debris in the microscar.

Bottom line: Peptides for skin care don't make scientific sense. The peptide piece of a protein is not as good at transmitting signals as the whole thing. Peptides are exposed to digestion on the skin surface and barriers to getting in. On the face of it, protein peptides are unlikely to work.

THE INSTANT FACE-LIFT PEPTIDES

Peptides are most often used in products that claim to reverse wrinkles. Some say they increase the skin support and others say they relax muscles like Botox. Let's take a look at the ones that have been put forward with a pseudoscientific justification and see whether there is any evidence to support their assertions.

Copper Peptides

Composed of three amino acids (glycine, histidine, and lysine) linked in a chain and wrapped around copper, this popular peptide was originally studied in wound healing, where it was applied to open wounds or injected with needles under the surface of the skin. Some of the published tests on animals show some promising effects in speeding wound repair. But these tests are far removed from rubbing a copper peptide onto intact facial skin to diminish wrinkles. Unfortunately, it is hard to find any scientific studies of copper peptide for anti-aging, beyond "data on file" notices on promotional Web sites.

Copper peptides are the key ingredient in the Neutrogena Visibly Firm Active Copper Peptide line.

The Faux Botox Peptides

In order to mimic the muscle-freezing properties of Botox, some potions state that they have peptides that relax the nerves to reverse wrinkles. Why, one ad for StriVectin even blares "Better than Botox?" despite the fact that no topical cream can ever be better than a product injected right into skin!

Dr. Kenneth R. Beer, a board-certified dermatologist, published a study[1] of seventy-seven women comparing StriVectin-SD, DDF Wrinkle Relax, and HydroDerm to Botox. He found that while every patient injected with Botox had a statistically significant improvement in wrinkles, none of the patients treated with any of the other three products had any improvement. In fact, the peptide creams were no different from the placebo.

Argireline (Acetyl Hexapeptide-3)

This peptide is supposed to interfere with a key protein inside the cell, called SNAP-25. The Botox toxin destroys SNAP-25 in nerve cells, which inhibits the release of the neurotransmitters sending signals from nerves to muscles. So, by analogy, says Lipotec, the Spanish manufacturer, their Argireline mimics the effects of Botox and inhibits the release of neurotransmitters. But the Botox toxin is specially produced by the *Botulinum* bacteria to enter only nerve cells and cut the SNAP-25 there—which is why Botox paralyzes nerves but does not affect other body functions.

Argireline is meant to be rubbed on all over the skin. If it really did penetrate into all kinds of cells, it would shut down SNAP-25 activity throughout the skin. If it really worked, no pigment would be made in your skin, turning it white; no sebum would be made, so your skin would turn dry and flake off; and your skin's immune defense against bacteria and viruses would collapse, leaving you vulnerable to massive infections.

Bear in mind, too, that Botox has to be injected with millimeter precision to avoid paralyzing the wrong muscles, like the ones that control your eyelids and cause your facial expressions. If this level of precision is required to inject a nerve agent, it's hardly believable that you could put a dab of a nerve-paralyzing peptide on your finger and rub it on over all the nerves of your face without disastrous consequences. (And wouldn't your finger get numb in the process?)

Among the products sold in the United States that contain Argireline are DDF Wrinkle Relax and Revlon Age Defying Makeup.

Eyeseryl

This is another peptide from Lipotec, the manufacturer of Argireline. Eyeseryl is intended to prevent glycation in skin. Glycation takes place when fructose, glucose, or another sugar binds uncontrollably to a protein or cell membrane. The glycation theory suggests that a diet high in sugar leads to advanced glycation end-products (AGE) in the skin, which disrupt the suppleness of the collagen and elastin network and cause wrinkles. Eyeseryl is found in WINspa Eyelift Cream and Episilk DCL Dark Circle Lightening Serum.

Glycation has been thoroughly studied in research with diabetics, who have high levels of circulating sugars. In fact, diabetic patients with high levels of AGE products go on to develop more serious consequences of the disease like retinopathy (eye disease) and nephropathy (kidney disease). However, the levels of AGE products in normal people, even the elderly, are much lower than those in diabetics and are not closely related to aging. As yet, no serious studies have shown that AGE products in normal people have any effect on wrinkles or any other health issue. Even if Eyeseryl worked to stop glycation in skin, which remains unproven, you don't need to worry about it in the first place.

Matrixyl

Composed of five linked amino acids that resemble a fragment of collagen, Matrixyl is a pentapeptide. Even Sederma, its manufacturer, admits that Matrixyl has no effect on nerves or muscles. So it is not a Botox alternative, despite the publicity craze fostered by StriVectin-SD, one of the products that contain Matrixyl.

Sederma states that these pieces of collagen somehow stimulate fibroblasts to make more collagen and thereby fix wrinkles—a claim that seems inconsistent with the most recent research. Remember, collagen fragments inhibit fibroblasts, they don't stimulate them. In fact, MMP-2 exists solely to remove this degraded collagen. The evidence supporting Matrixyl remains unpublished, while Dr. Beer's study cited previously showed that it had no effect.

In addition to StriVectin-SD, Matrixyl is also a key ingredient in Olay's Regenerist Daily Regenerating Serum.

Polypeptide 153

The height of bombastic marketing nonsense was reached by Voss Laboratories (the same people behind StriVectin) with their product Amatokin. The key ingredient is polypeptide 153, which they say was developed in a Russian high-security lab and is supposed to stimulate the skin's stem cells. There's not a scrap of scientific evidence to back this up, and it is implausible to reputable scientists. The company has tried to generate controversy about its product using the stem cell debate, buttressed with "secret" Hollywood admirers, in an attempt to make bad news into good sales. Don't fall for it.

Bottom line: Peptides are not all they are cracked up to be; in fact, they seem to be the latest in a long string of cosmetic fads that make no scientific sense and have little or no evidence to support them. Objective clinical studies suggest these products are nothing more than moisturizers.

MORE WRINKLE MYTHS

Ingredients other than peptides have been shamelessly promoted as wrinkle cures without any scientific evidence. Here are some of the more popular botanical extracts and chemicals and what we know about them scientifically.

Boswelox

You probably know boswellia resin as its derivative, the spice frankincense. Boswellia has been long valued as an anti-inflammatory agent, and animal studies have shown its potential for reducing joint and intestinal inflammation. However, the scientific literature has no reference to boswellia as a muscle relaxant or a wrinkle reducer in the skin.

You wouldn't know that if you saw the ad for the L'Oréal's Wrinkle De-Crease series. "A breakthrough phyto-complex," is how they describe this concentrated dose of boswellia extract and manganese. This is said to assist in reducing the appearance of lines caused by "facial micro-contractions." Eighty percent of users instantly saw smoother skin, according to the packaging literature.

We tested in our laboratory the ability of this product to alter nerve sensations, which we would have expected if Boswelox really dampened the nerves that cause muscle contraction. However, despite repeated applications, we were unable to detect a change in the nerve response in skin using a sensitive machine that measures nerve perception. Across the Atlantic, in response to criticisms from the United Kingdom's advertising regulator, L'Oréal in Britain has agreed to modify some of the claims it makes about Boswelox.

DMAE (Dimethylaminoethanol)

This naturally occurring substance, chemically similar to the B vitamin choline, has been shown in some studies where it was taken orally to enhance cognitive ability and memory among the elderly and to offer a modest increase in the lifespan of some animals. It does stimulate nerve cells to release acetylcholine, a neurotransmitter. DMAE has been sold in Europe as a nutritional supplement for some neurological disorders, but no reliable evidence shows that it works in any disease.

Some have called DMAE an "instant face-lift," but the explanation for why that's so is a bit convoluted. DMAE supposedly stimulates the nerves to cause muscles to contract, producing a "face-lift" effect and reducing wrinkles. But wait a minute! Botox is a well-documented *relaxer* of facial muscles. How can wrinkles be removed by both relaxing (Botox) and contracting (DMAE) muscles in the face?

Johnson & Johnson, which markets DMAE in Neutrogena Advanced Solutions, has reported that its studies with 3 percent DMAE produced mixed results, with some measurements of an increase in skin firmness. In our lab we tested the ability of this DMAE product to alter nerve sensations using a sensitive measuring device called a neurometer. Despite an application to the skin of volunteers at night and an application the following morning, no change in nerve response was measured. There don't seem to be any serious studies to support the action of this ingredient in skin.

Some aspects of DMAE in skin have been patented by Dr. Nicholas Perricone, and many N.V. Perricone M.D. products contain it—including the Neuropeptide Facial Conformer (for the whopping price of $570), the Body Toning Lotion, and the Active Tinted Moisturizer. This ingredient also appears in Source Naturals Skin Eternal Cream as well as Reviva Labs Alpha Lipoic Acid, Vitamin C Ester, and DMAE Hand and Body Lotion.

Bottom line: DMAE is an ingredient in some very expensive lotions, but no reliable evidence shows that it works.

GABA (Gamma-Aminobutyric Acid)

Produced in the body and classified as a neurotransmitter, this amino acid appears in such creams as Freeze 24-7 products (whose motto is "Nature. Not Needles") and Dr. Brandt Crease Release. GABA is touted to reduce muscle-fiber activity and diminish the appearance of fine lines and wrinkles "within minutes" by causing a "freeze" of nerves controlling facial muscles—just like Botox. It has the same problems as the peptides—the explanation is not plausible and the supporting evidence is lacking. We tested Freeze 24-7 with the neurometer to see if it would indeed reduce nerve sensation. In fact, we got the complete opposite result—Freeze 24-7 actually was a mild irritant that aggravated nerve endings!

It's true that some of these products do produce an immediate smoothing effect—but the secret ingredient here may well be one of a number of simple polymers that acts as temporary glue on the skin. After applying it to skin the water evaporates, and the abundant but now-dry polymer contracts to give an immediate tightening sensation. This dried polymer may also explain the warning on the Freeze 24-7 package insert that "a light white residue can appear after absorption if you have dry skin."

The polymer rubs off in less than an hour, returning your skin to its normal, pre–Freeze 24-7 state.

Bottom line: The evidence for the antiwrinkle effect of GABA is no better than for peptides or DMAE, and it makes no more sense, either. The effects have to do with the drying effects of the lotion rather than any real effect of GABA on wrinkles.

MMP Inhibitors

Many new products, such as the Patricia Wexler M.D. skin-care line with MMPi, and Dr. Matthew Galumbeck's Skin Amnesty line with col- hibin (hydrolized rice protein), sound alarm bells with me. Same goes for butcher's broom rhizone (*Ruscus aculeatus*) or special soy peptides. All of these products fall under the category of general MMP inhibitors.

As we discussed, MMPs are a group of enzymes that pave the way for healing by degrading shredded collagen and elastin around a wound site. One in particular, MMP-1, seems to be turned on by sunlight and to cause wrinkles. But some MMPs, like MMP-2 and MMP-9, are valu- able to the skin in clearing away the normal debris and keeping fibro- blasts pumping out collagen. Therefore, inhibiting *all* MMPs is probably not a good idea, since you need MMP-2 and MMP-9. You might, over time, actually turn normal skin into photoaged skin. Today's MMP in- hibitors, however, don't differentiate among the various MMP enzymes.

A better way to stop MMPs might be to cut them off before they start—by toning down inflammation in the skin, which is a signal to cells for their release. A multitasking moisturizer with anti-inflammatory botanicals such as chamomile, aloe, or evodia extract can help.

Bottom line: MMP inhibitors should be more finely tuned before being used to stop wrinkles. The products sound scientific but the kinks have not yet been worked out, and they are not recommended.

TGF-Beta

Products with TGF-beta claim to stimulate cell division and thicken the skin with healthy, growing cells that fill in wrinkles. TGF-beta is a powerful cell-signaling protein with drastic effects on cells, including acting as a trigger for scleroderma, a disease that causes hardening of organs throughout the body. It is also a major player in wound healing, in ways we are only beginning to understand. One thing for sure is that it slows up or stops cell division (exactly the opposite of what its proponents say it's supposed to do). Therefore, applying it to the skin doesn't seem like such a good idea.

Like Botox, TGF-beta is so potent that smearing it over the face might have cataclysmic consequences—if there really was enough in the formula and if it was actually able to penetrate into skin, neither of which is true. There is no reliable research support for applying it to skin for wrinkles.

TGF-beta appears in the Jan Marini Skin Research Transformation Serum and TNS Recovery Complex from SkinMedica.

Bottom line: Products with TGF-beta are not recommended.

HOW TO USE WRINKLE CREAMS

As we have seen, no one miracle ingredient exists to remove or otherwise "cure" wrinkles. There are, however, products that greatly reduce fine lines and wrinkles and fill out and brighten skin. Combined with sun protection and repair, you can experience a definite improvement. Just keep your expectations real.

The best way to diminish wrinkles is to use products with synergis-

Lip Plumping

Full, plump lips have become such a rage that a new phrase—"trout pout"—was coined to describe the formerly thin lips of Hollywood stars that had suddenly morphed into enormous smackers.

The most effective (and most expensive) way to achieve puffed-up lips is with the use of injectible fillers, such as hyaluronic acid (Restylane), collagen, or fat. These aren't permanent, so injections need to be repeated every six months or so.

Cosmetic plumpers are a lot easier on the lips and your pocketbook, although they barely last a few hours. Bearing names like Joey New York Super Duper Lips, Girl Cosmetics Lip Enhancing Lip Gloss, DuWop Lip Venom, Sally Hansen Lip Inflation, and Lierac Coherence Lip Contour Fixing Care, they're applied in stick, gel, or cream form.

Sounds great, right? Well, lip plumpers work by causing irritation—with some of the ingredients like mint, peppermint, and menthol that I suggested you avoid in chapter 3. And this irritated lip tissue swells. This is easy to accomplish, since lips have no protective outer layer (explaining why they dry out so easily).

Many manufacturers warn customers to expect a tingle. That can be a real understatement. Some of them hurt, a lot. That said, there is no evidence of lasting damage. It's up to you to decide whether the irritation and pain are worth having slightly bigger lips for a few hours of face time.

tically designed ingredients in the morning and in the evening. The regimen that follows has four easy steps that take no more than a minute or two. Always let each layer dry down before applying a new cream.

MORNING REGIMEN

Every morning, follow these steps. A good multitasking product will combine more than one of these steps, so you may need to use only two products in your morning routine. Recommendations for specific products can be found in chapter 13.

1. Cleanse your skin, gently. Use warm water alone if possible.

2. Moisturize with a multitasking product. An optimal moisturizer will include vitamins C and E to build the collagen layers, an ingredient like ursolic acid to strengthen the top barrier layer, and a calming ingredient to reduce inflammation.

3. Reprogram DNA and encourage DNA repair and recovery with key nutrients.

4. Brighten to even out skin tone. This is an optional step that need not be done every day. It can be done during the time that you are also exfoliating at night. If you do use brighteners, always apply a sunscreen before going out.

5. Protect with sunscreen with an SPF of at least 15. Use a higher SPF if you have fair skin.

EVENING REGIMEN

1. Cleanse your skin thoroughly to remove makeup and excess oil.

2. Moisturize with a multitasking product. An optimal moisturizer will contain vitamins C and E and encourage DNA reprogramming and repair.

3. Alternate exfoliation and retinol treatment
   Use an AHA/PHA exfoliation cream nightly for six weeks.
   Then use a retinol or retinoic acid (prescription) cream for
     six weeks.
   Repeat the cycle, using each product for six weeks.

ELEVEN

The Doctor Treatments

It's an understatement to say that many of the new, noninvasive cosmetic procedures done by skilled dermatologists or plastic surgeons can have a dramatic effect on the shape of your face and the texture and appearance of your skin. In fact, these procedures are now so popular, and so much a part of the mainstream, that women often proudly boast of the discomfort they've endured (while flashing a bruise or two) and the thousands of dollars they've spent because the results can be so pleasing.

On the other hand, the results can be so overdone that some women end up with frozen, expressionless faces, cheeks with angles not known to nature, and lips so puffy you fear they'll split open with a smile.

A decade or so ago, deep chemical peels or face-lifts were the treatment of choice for women of a certain age who found themselves with drooping and sagging skin, but there were serious drawbacks. A deep peel was incredibly painful and necessitated a long recuperation process and produced skin so raw and oozing that venturing out of the house was not an option. And a face-lift is not a minor operation; it must be done under general anesthesia, by a surgeon with the skill of a sculptor, and the recuperation process is long and painful. Nor were these inexpensive propositions. A deep peel shouldn't have to be repeated, but contrary to popular belief, a face-lift is not forever. Gravity still takes its toll, after all. Faces elongate over time, the skin becomes thinner, and new folds arise—especially if you don't stay out of the sun!

A face-lift can also never do one important thing: It can't replace lost volume. As we age, the fat that once padded our baby cheeks disappears. And since face-lifts cut and pull, anyone worried about looking gaunt could end up looking, well, unnaturally *stretched*.

Enter the injectable fillers, which are far less invasive, and as a result have transformed the natural aging process as they instantly replace lost volume, subtly plumping up faces and filling in wrinkles. They can't be used all over the face, though, which is where Botox comes in. Derived from a toxin, Botox relaxes and freezes muscles so that wrinkles slacken and new ones don't form. And then lasers, chemical peels, and light treatments can tackle the texture of the skin itself.

Botox and fillers are as close to a genuine wrinkle cure as we can get at the moment. But they are, of course, *of* the moment. They don't last. Eventually, the body recovers from Botox's muscle-paralyzing effect, and filler substances are gradually reabsorbed and harmlessly excreted. Which can be a good thing if you weren't happy with the results. Or a bad thing when you get the bill, which can start with a few hundred dollars for a single injection. To get a face full of filler by one of the top dermatologists in New York or Beverly Hills can easily set you back five figures, depending on how many syringes you need. None of these procedures is covered by health insurance, and you're going to need to go back within four to six months. The average consumer can hardly afford such an expensive treatment plan over a long period of time.

As temporarily effective and increasingly popular as these new treatments are, despite their hefty price tag, they do *not* reprogram the skin. They don't do anything to repair your DNA. They are fine to do if you care to spend all that money on a temporary quick fix. They're safe, personalized solutions to aging concerns. But they're not a replacement for the daily regimen using products created in the New Skin-Care Revolution that can bring about a true reprogramming of skin to reconstruct and maintain your beauty for decades to come.

Let's take a look at the most popular procedures.

BOTOX

Botox is amazing, among the first wave of products in the New Skin-Care Revolution. Who would have thought that a neurotoxin would freeze the foreheads of Hollywood?

Botox is the FDA-approved brand name for the toxin derived from botulinum toxin type A, the same substance that causes deadly botulism poisoning from tainted food. When diluted and injected, this toxin paralyzes nerves so that they can no longer direct muscles to contract. It takes a few days for the full effect to kick in, but once it does, wrinkles literally disappear. Botox usually lasts for four to six months and gradually wears off. Those who have regular, repeated treatments often find that wrinkles formed from use—on the forehead from frowning or near the eyes and lips from squinting or pursing—often aren't as prominent when they do reappear. Since Botox prevents you from using these muscles, the muscles themselves aren't overtaxed and skin stays smoother longer.

Botox's wide popularity as a wrinkle remover lies not only in its potency, but also in its subtlety. In an instant, it can lift an eyebrow by paralyzing the muscle between the brow ridge and the eye sockets. It also goes to work controlling the facial muscles that squeeze the skin into the ridges and furrows that create permanent creasing between the brows, known as glabellar lines. (Botox was, actually, originally FDA approved only for use on the glabellar lines.) Since faces contain dozens of muscles, many contours, clefts, and channels can be sculpted and smoothed with the careful use of just one syringe full of Botox.

Although millions of Botox injections are given each year, the procedure is far from trivial, and great skill is needed in performing it. The face is dense with hundreds of muscle pairs. They may be only a few millimeters in width, a few centimeters in length, and buried under other crisscrossing muscles. Some muscles control nonvital facial expressions, but many keep the eyelids from drooping, the lips from sagging, and allow the mouth to form into a circle to pronounce a vocabulary of words. And, of course, to open up to let you eat! A thorough knowledge of anatomy—

as well as a trained aesthetic eye—is a prerequisite for anyone sticking a narrow needle into this haystack of muscles and making wrinkles disappear.

In the right hands, Botox can be injected in many more areas than the forehead. It can erase crow's feet, lift the corners of the lips, and ease jowls and skin bands in the neck. A drop under the nose can even lift drooping cartilage.

In the wrong hands, however, Botox can leave you with, paradoxically, a drooping forehead and paralyzed eyelids and lips.

It does seem, however, that some consumers are choosing to be overinjected, so that their foreheads become as smooth as a baby's bottom, leaving them unable to have any range of expression in their faces. It is not only a telltale giveaway but can be pretty scary. Faces paralyzed with Botox may benefit poker players and runway models, but the rest of us, whether we know it or not, rely on visual clues from one another's faces to convey meaning in even the most trivial of conversations. Many of these cues are subtle. What would the art of flirtation be without the barely perceptible lift of an eyebrow?

And we may be hardwired with a basic human need to use all our facial muscles in order to be expressive. Just think of how often you smile or frown or laugh or grimace when you're on the phone or alone in your office or at home. The world's first face-transplant patient, Isabelle Dinoire, emphasized this point several months after her surgery in 2005. The most satisfying aspect of her transplant was, as she remarked, "being able to show emotions through my face."

The next generation of Botox is around the corner. Slated for imminent approval are Dysport and Reloxin, other forms of botulinum toxin that last slightly longer. Coming down the pike is Merz's Xeomin, and Mentor's Puretox, new forms of the neurotoxin for wrinkle treatment that are more highly purified and less likely to produce allergic reactions.

Bottom line: Botox is a very effective, if expensive, wrinkle fix. It requires repeat injections every four to six months. Its popularity attests to how well it works, but choose a respected and responsible doctor; in the wrong hands it can be overdone and result in the frozen look.

PEELS

CHEMICAL PEELS

Exfoliating with chemicals can be done much more aggressively in the dermatologist's office than it can be done at home. AHAs that can be sold over the counter at only 10 percent are available at your physician's office at up to 30 percent; other acids, like TCA (trichloroacetic acid), can be used only at the doctor's office in solutions of 15 to 50 percent, and phenol in solutions of up to 88 percent.

These acid formulations essentially dissolve the upper layer of skin (light to medium peels) and, in the case of TCA and phenol, partially destroy the lower dermal layer (medium to deep peels). This wound stimulates collagen growth, and once the skin has healed, the new layers are fresh and smooth.

TCA is also used on the throat and other parts of the body where phenol cannot be used, and, unlike phenol, does not require anesthesia. (In fact, the TCA itself acts as a local anesthesia.) Phenol peels, the deepest and most severe of them all, produce a more dramatic and long-lasting effect than the others, but anyone who's had one will tell you how excruciatingly painful they can be.

Phenol peels are rarely done anymore, as they were tricky to control and were also associated with cardiac complications. Most dermatologists prefer to use high-concentration AHAs or Jessner's peel (made from salicylic acid, lactic acid, and resorcinol).

Bottom line: Peels in the doctor's office are an intensified form of what can be achieved at home. Nevertheless, for many the AHA/BHA/PHA home treatments are completely satisfactory, as is shown by the widespread drop in the number of peeling procedures done by dermatologists.

LIQUID NITROGEN

Instead of peeling a whole face when only a small area is overly pigmented, liquid nitrogen can be dabbed on or sprayed on to freeze the skin down to the layer with the melanin to remove it, producing what looks like a burn. Over the next few days, a scab forms, and it will peel

away in about a week, leaving clear, new skin in its place. If done properly, the procedure works well. However, the colored spot often makes
a gradual return over the course of several months, and a new round of
freezing is required.

In some cases, though, the new skin may be even lighter than the
surrounding skin, and if the whole spot is not covered with liquid nitrogen, a halo of pigment can be left behind. This treatment is recommended for small age spots resistant to treatment with brighteners.

MICRODERMABRASION

The principle of inducing a wound-healing response in the skin without
making a wound lies behind many of the innovations in anti-aging skin
care. Mechanical exfoliants, such as scrubbing grains and microdermabrasion, are less effective than peels at disrupting the top layers of
skin and invoking a repair response, but they are far less painful. As with
peels, new collagen will be stimulated and skin will look younger and
smoother.

Microdermabrasion done by a dermatologist involves the use of a
machine that spews small sandlike grains to polish the skin. A powerful
vacuum immediately sucks up the grains, allowing for greater control of
the depth of peeling. This procedure has largely supplanted the older
dermabrasion technique, in which a rotating wire brush brutally annihi-
lated all skin in its path. Microdermabrasion is recommended for people with mild photoaging and those who want a quick "tune-up" before
an event. Be sure to leave a few days for recovery as the skin tends to be
pink and slightly tender immediately afterward.

The initial treatment may be spread over two or three sessions, with
maintenance treatments every three to six months. Don't forget to restore the antioxidant reservoir removed by this procedure with a good vitamin A, C, and E product.

IPL (INTENSE PULSED LIGHT)

The IPL device delivers high-energy bursts of light to the skin. Similar
to but not quite a laser, it is far less likely to burn or darken skin the way

lasers can. It's primarily used to remove unwanted hair and tattoos and destroy blood vessels that cause spider veins. When it comes to wrinkle treatments, this is a sledgehammer solution for a problem that only needs a tinker. That's because the IPL is destructive, and wrinkle treatment needs a gentler approach, with only the stimulation of the wound-healing response. Therefore, the IPL should be used to address specific and local problems, rather than for face resurfacing, which could require excessive recovery time.

INJECTABLE FILLERS

While Botox can smooth some savage wrinkles, it can't, as you know by now, be injected all over the face. Only the most skilled dermatologists dare inject it near the eyes or lips. But Botox is only one type of injectable, and a filler is another. They are completely different substances and have different functions. Botox is meant to smooth wrinkles that come from muscles being used. Fillers are meant to replace lost volume.

Fillers are composed of thick but inert materials that, when injected, literally fill in crevices and depressions, smoothing out surfaces. The most popular fillers are either your own body's fat, removed from the hips or buttocks, or materials made from collagen or cross-linked hyaluronic acid to form microscopic grains that vary in consistency and tensile strength. Slightly different kinds of grains are used for different kinds of creases and wrinkles. Some are better suited to fine, surface wrinkles, while others can tackle deeper creases and lines. Side effects of fillers are usually minor, with pain at the injection site, bruising, tenderness, swelling, and redness being the most common.

Fillers work right away, although it may be hard to see results for a few days as many patients tend to get a bit swollen and bruised. A few sessions are often needed for optimal results, and tune-ups every three to twelve months are required to maintain the look. Fillers are made from natural materials compatible with the body to avoid allergic reactions, so they're subject to the body's natural turnover processes, including digestion and absorption. Thus, they degrade over the course of three to six months, eventually disappearing entirely.

Injecting a filler may have an unintended benefit in photoaged skin, if Dr. John Voorhees of the University of Michigan is right. He has hypothesized that in photoaged skin—where supporting structures have been chewed to debris by chomping enzymes—the fibroblast cells stop making collagen when they lose their anchoring. When fillers are injected into sun-damaged skin, they may well give these desperate skin cells something to hold on to. This would then allow the cells to turn on their own natural collagen production to finish the job for the fillers, which would last a lot longer.

Not all fillers are the same, and it is important to recognize the different types and their advantages and disadvantages before agreeing to any procedure. Let's take a look at the three most common kinds of fillers.

COLLAGEN

The first fillers were made from collagen and are still widely used in two forms, called Zyderm and Zyplast. They're both derived from cow collagen, and both contain lidocaine to deaden the pain after injection. Zyderm is more malleable than Zyplast and is injected just under the skin surface to fill in fine wrinkles and acne scars. Zyplast is made by cross-linking the bovine collagen fibers to form tougher cables that are injected deeper into the dermis to fill deeper lines, furrows, and scars. Large areas can actually be sculpted by layering Zyderm over Zyplast to achieve finely textured changes. Zyplast is also commonly used to plump lips—when it is overused or misused here, the patient can end up with the notorious "trout pout."

A major drawback to these fillers is that some patients are allergic to bovine collagen, so all candidates must be pretested for allergies. A tiny sample is injected into the forearm and then evaluated two to three weeks afterward and then again four weeks later for signs of redness, inflammation, or itching. The testing is usually repeated on the other arm and observed for two weeks. If all goes well, the procedure can begin about six weeks after the first skin test.

Collagen fillers are tried and true, and affordable, but the allergic potential and relatively short time before a repeat injection is needed (less than five months) make them the least desirable of the fillers.

Alternatives to bovine collagen are the newer CosmoDerm and CosmoPlast, made from human collagen. The body recognizes this human collagen as "self" and doesn't produce an immune response, so allergy pretesting is not needed. CosmoDerm and CosmoPlast are also composed of unlinked and cross-linked collagen, respectively, and have the same functions as Zyderm and Zyplast. Soon to come is collagen made by biotechnology, such as the genetically engineered one from FibroGen, as well as from Isolagen, which is a collagen created from the patient's own skin cells, cultured in a laboratory. These are all more expensive than the standard collagen fillers.

HYALURONIC ACID

Another group of fillers is made from hyaluronic acid, a long-chain sugar formed naturally in the body. The cross-linked chains have tough, elastic properties that make them quite suitable as fillers. None of them needs to be allergy pretested. They tend to last from five to six months; the more injections you have over time, the longer they may last.

One type of hyaluronic acid filler, Hylaform, is made from the comb on the head of roosters, and its soft character makes it the perfect choice for lip augmentation. Restylane is made from hyaluronic acid purified from fermented bacteria (not the infection-causing kind!). Similar in structure to Hylaform, Restylane is widely used for plumping lips, adding volume to the cheeks, and filling in the nasolabial fold, the groove running from the side of the nose to the side of the mouth. Captique, a nonanimal hyaluronic acid gel, has been approved for severe wrinkles and folds.

The lack of immunologic reaction makes hyaluronic acid fillers the first choice for many doctors. They can be easily and evenly delivered and distributed into creases and folds and last longer than collagen.

POLY-L-LACTIC ACID

Sculptra is poly-L-lactic acid formed into injectable microparticles. It was originally approved for restoring fullness in the faces of HIV patients wasted by the disease but is now being used off-label for cosmetic procedures. It is used in thicker skin and is not recommended for lips or around the eyes. Repeated injections may be required until the desired look is achieved, but once it is, it can last for one to two years, giving it a notable advantage.

FILLERS OF THE FUTURE

With millions of procedures performed each year, the demand for injectables has become an astounding phenomenon. Huge corporate acquisition battles are waged over the companies making these fillers, which has spurred them to find new substances that have varying degrees of thickness, making them more versatile, and that last longer than the typical four to six months. Expect to see a steady stream of new fillers over the next few years. On the horizon is a newer form of hyaluronic acid called Juvéderm, with very small particles that make it less likely to produce side effects, as well as Radiesse, made from calcium hydroxylapatite and originally used in reconstructive dentistry. Others, including Evolence, a new collagen from Colbar Ltd., are also in the pipeline. If you consider them, discuss with your doctor three things: (1) their potential for allergic reaction or other side effects; (2) how long before they are reabsorbed and the injection must be repeated; (3) the cost for a whole treatment (not just a single injection or one session).

Bottom line: The preferred filler today for moderate photoaging and wrinkles is made from hyaluronic acid, but new products are on the way, so stay tuned. You should expect a filler not to cause allergic reactions and to last at least five months. Even severe wrinkles and loss of fat can be treated with the appropriate filler.

LASERS AND OTHER LIGHT TREATMENTS

Offering a high-tech means of exfoliation and peeling, the newest generation of lasers has also become very big business for dermatologists, plastic surgeons, and salons. The goal, as with other exfoliation technologies, is to peel the upper layers of the skin and trigger a wound-healing response that rejuvenates collagen and rebuilds the upper epidermal skin layer. The laser light is absorbed by different components of the skin, which then heat up and are destroyed. By using different colors of light, a laser can be literally directed to treat different depths of the skin.

Because they are so precise, lasers have a decided advantage over the less easily controlled chemical peels. The design of a laser device determines how much energy is used and where the beam of light is directed, so the depth of the damage is pinpointed. This way, practitioners can literally dial in the degree of peeling to be achieved. Many species of lasers are on the market, and each one has a specific function. Pigment lasers correct discoloration, while resurfacing lasers remove the sluggish skin tone that comes from buildup in the stratum corneum, restore a smooth surface, and spur new collagen growth in lower levels of the dermis.

All this high technology comes with a price, however. The lasers themselves are expensive, and the treatments aren't cheap, either. Most require a long course of treatments spaced over several months for optimal results.

Don't forget that lasers are dangerous in the wrong hands. They can burn skin and produce wide swatches of discolored skin that are very difficult if not impossible to treat. Plus, the wide array of lasers (and other light sources) can be intimidating. The best solution is to select a dermatologist or plastic surgeon with a variety of laser and laserlike choices in his or her practice—and have a serious evaluation before choosing a treatment. You are putting yourself at risk if you choose to go to a physician-supervised salon where a technician with limited experience does the work. Be sure that the person wielding the device has extensive experience with that particular laser.

No laser is a miracle cure, but if you have reasonable expectations, you can see a definite improvement in your skin tone as well as fewer wrinkles.

Bottom line: Lasers have the advantage of quick and specific treatment. Many types of lasers are used, and new ones are on the way. Choose a treatment office that offers different choices and discuss with a well-trained physician which option is best for you.

Here is a review of some of the most widely used lasers:

CO$_2$ (CARBON DIOXIDE) LASERS

CO$_2$ lasers are widely used to treat the upper layer and some of the lower layers of the skin. They work well but they are not for minimal wrinkles, as pain and oozing can follow, and the treated area looks fairly hideous for several weeks afterward. The skin can also lose its pigment. This type of laser is recommended only for moderate to serious photoaging and deeper wrinkles.

FRAXEL SR LASER

The Fraxel SR laser causes fewer side effects than the CO_2 laser by delivering microscopic light beams that dot the skin with pinpricks that extend into the dermis, where they can stimulate collagen growth. The idea is that the tissue surrounding the pinprick areas, known as micro thermal zones, survives intact, contributing healthy cells and growth factors to the traumatized areas. This treatment still requires local anesthesia and a total of three to five sessions spaced five to seven days apart, but only a little downtime is involved, as the skin's surface looks normal throughout the series of treatments. A competing device, the ProFractional, promises more precise energy delivery, meaning fewer treatments; time will tell if this is truly an improvement. Overall, the Fraxel technique is the recommended procedure for treating minimal and moderate photoaging and the beginning of wrinkles.

TITAN LASER

The Titan uses an infrared light device (not really a laser) to heat the skin and contract collagen. A cooling coil keeps the upper layers from overheating, while the infrared rays travel deeper into the dermis to shrink the collagen and tighten the skin. The principle is the same as the radio-frequency devices described below, and the benefits are also modest, with the same risk of pain and release of collagen-degrading enzymes (which may in the end be counterproductive). Until more clinical evidence supports this treatment, it is not recommended as the first choice.

RADIOFREQUENCY DEVICES

Radiofrequency devices don't produce focused beams of light like lasers do; instead, they use radio frequencies, the energy delivered by waves in

Lasers and Lightening

Since lasers literally vaporize the unwanted pigment granules buried in the skin, you'd think they'd be extremely promising for the treatment of hyperpigmentation. Unfortunately, their results for many colors of skin spots have generally been disappointing, and lasers like the alexandrite 755 nm are still considered more of a backup treatment should topical treatments fail.

The problem when it comes to treating pigmentation is that these lasers also induce a wound-healing response—which always includes some degree of inflammation—that can often leave darker skin tones even darker than before. Lasers work best on lighter skin with darker spots and not vice versa. This is hugely frustrating, of course, for those with darker skin who need treatment yet fear potential results that could actually be worse than the original condition.

A new generation of light sources, such as the Apogee Elite, combining green light with infrared, claim to be able to treat even the darkest skin tones. Their reported success, however, is more clear-cut when it comes to treating acne scarring without leaving a hyperpigmented spot behind. So far, they're not very effective at clearing melasma or other color spots in people of color. Hopefully, as laser technology improves, we'll be seeing lasers that can treat all skin tones with equal success.

the range of radio signals, to destroy the upper and some of the lower skin layers. They also claim to use heat to "tighten" skin. There is really no distinct advantage in these treatments when compared to lasers, as the resulting tissue closely resembles laser-treated skin. The two main radiofrequency devices in use are covered here.

PORTRAIT PSR 3 HIGH-ENERGY PLASMA DEVICE

The Portrait PSR 3 high-energy plasma device generates heat using ul-tra–high frequency radio waves to convert nitrogen gas into millisecond pulses of heat. With a single pass of the instrument head over the skin, a burst of heat is sent into the treatment area. The high temperature is quickly dissipated outward by the upper layers of skin, but at the lower layers the heat keeps traveling deeper. The result is that the device heats the underlying dermis without immediately damaging the epidermis. The skin covering the treatment site remains in place while the wound-healing response begins underneath. The PSR treatment is approved for wrinkles, superficial skin damage, and precancerous spots and actinic keratoses.

There is a flip side, however. At the level of energy needed to produce real results, the upper skin darkens and sheds in about three days, and the skin stays red for another two or three days. The heating is painful, and local anesthesia or sometimes even oral painkillers are used. Several treatments are needed, and collagen deposits may take several months to form, while tissue remodeling may go on for an even longer period.

VISAGE THERMACOOL RADIOFREQUENCY DEVICE

The ThermaCool radiofrequency device by Visage uses radio waves to tighten the skin. It works by heating the skin, which causes the rods of collagen in the bottom layer to contract and stiffen the supporting tissue. The danger is that too much heating of the skin can also cause release of enzymes that degrade collagen, so be careful. The proper course of treatment is several passes of the radio-frequency device emitting low energy over the treatment site, rather than a single pass of higher energy.

Unfortunately, this heating of the skin is uncomfortable, and topical anesthesia often doesn't do much to numb the pain. The treatment is not nearly as effective as a face-lift.

Bottom line: Radiofrequency devices are not a miracle advance over lasers. They have the disadvantage of generating heat, which is painful and may induce collagen-digesting enzymes, and the benefits are no better than the alternatives. This seems like a technology in search of a treatment, and it is not recommended.

TWELVE

The Future of Skin Care

Over the last few years, there have been many remarkable changes in the way science has tackled skin-care needs. Even more are in the pipeline, so let's take a look at what you can expect to see on your shelves in the future.

BOTANICALS—CAPTURING THE ESSENCE

Botanicals can be a wonder. They smell great, are evocative of luxurious pampering—bathing in water strewn with flower petals or getting massaged with fragrant oils—and skin-care science is now able to identify many of their active components. That's good news for consumers. Once specific molecular structures become known, these essences can either be purified directly from the plants or synthesized and purified to perfection in a chemistry lab.

Being able to synthesize these botanical extracts is an amazing accomplishment. Not only does it allow us to use them at higher concentrations than are found in nature so their effect is more potent, but it also gives us a consistent and dependable source. Lab-created bio-identical essences will also greatly lessen any unwanted side effects or allergic reactions triggered by impurities in unrefined potions.

As techniques improve, we'll also see many more secrets uncovered from plants, especially through exploring folk medicines that have centuries of use attesting to their safety and by being able, in the lab, to sift through hundreds of thousands of compounds to look for special bioactivity. Best of all, we won't have to chop down the Amazon rain forest to enjoy the benefits of its exotic flora.

When you are serious about skin care, you welcome the day when the packaging lists exactly what chemical is in the product that is producing the result you are looking for. As long as you accept feel-good phrases like "watermelon extract" and "pomegranate juice" as a sufficient description, you will have hype, misleading labels, confusion, and products that don't work.

Bottom line: In the next few years, look for new botanically based products with purified and standardized ingredients yielding better results and fewer allergic or irritant reactions than ever before.

COSMETIC COMPANIES VERSUS DERMATOLOGISTS

A decade or so ago, dermatologists weren't exactly high-profile physicians. Oh, sure, they tackled serious problems like skin cancer and acne, but needing to visit one wasn't exactly something that thrilled most patients. Now, of course, with the advent of injectable fillers and Botox, along with chemical peels, microdermabrasion, and lasers, seeing a cosmetic dermatologist or plastic surgeon regularly has become a must for millions of women who are excited with how much better they can now look. Top doctors in major cities have waiting lists several months long.

Many dermatologists have also gotten even more serious about giving their patients more than in-office care and have formulated their own take-home product lines. At first these dermatologist-driven lines were priced at the level of prestige cosmetics. But with the demand for cosmeceuticals showing no sign of abating, even mass-market drugstores like CVS have jumped into the world of skin care with their own moderately priced and dermatologist-branded skin-care offerings. A growing number of products are also addressing long-unmet medical concerns, like acne, and continue to focus on new challenges, like rosacea.

One huge influence that medicine has had on skin care is the shift in focus to prevention. Just as we've become able to recognize important markers of heart disease, like hypertension and high cholesterol, before any signs appear—which has greatly reduced the death rate from coronary disease—so are consumers finally beginning to get the message about the effects of sunlight on aging and skin health. Women in their twenties and thirties are becoming as conscious of sun protection as those in their forties and fifties, and we have hope that there may be declining rates of skin disease and cancer if the use of sun protection becomes more widespread at an earlier age. As the benefits for prevention become more widely appreciated, consumers will be motivated to start buying better skin-care products that deliver genuine prevention and improvement. The quick cosmetic fix so beloved by many today will be nudged aside to make room for investment treatments that perform over the long haul.

Cosmetics and medicine may soon join forces in other ways. Many of the 12 million cosmetic procedures performed by dermatologists and plastic surgeons each year—from laser treatments to face-lifts—provoke a wound-healing response or involve a lengthy recuperation after surgery. New skin-care products that stimulate recuperation, as well as lessen pain, swelling, and bruising, will help many patients get better and look better sooner.

Bottom line: Dermatologists and plastic surgeons are in high demand, and cosmetic companies are competing with them for clients. Even drugstores are launching upscale products to attract these customers. All this attention will push skin care toward prevention of problems and procedures combined with topicals for faster results.

GENETIC COSMETICS

Understanding DNA's role in skin regulation has already brought us to the brink of gene therapy for skin. One way is to use a synthetic bit of decoy DNA to derail the gene activation pathway early on, sending it to a harmless dead end—which should reduce redness, irritation, and sensitivity. Another way is to use a piece of DNA to trick the cell into stepping up its repair activities. Gene therapy for skin is still in its experimental stages, but being able to manipulate DNA may totally change skin care in the near future.

What's also exciting to think about is how our improved knowledge of DNA and skin care will lead to truly personalized skin care. The Human Genome Project has not only listed every gene in human DNA, but it has also given us the tools to examine each of those genes in any individual. Ten years ago, such a probing examination would have cost thousands of dollars and months of work. Today, hundreds of genes can be examined in about two weeks for two dollars per gene. In the future, the test will be done at a cosmetic counter while you wait and will be so inexpensive that stores will give it away for free with every purchase!

While we all have the same set of genes, each gene comes in different flavors for each individual. A single change in the coding sequence in DNA may have no effect, a minor effect, or a disastrous effect, such as birth defects or miscarriages. DNA changes without any effects or with minor effects are known as gene polymorphisms, from *poly*, meaning "many," and *morphs*, meaning "forms." Gene polymorphisms determine hair and skin color. Blond hair is a polymorphism, for example; it's a very minor polymorphism in the gene pool of most of Africa but the dominant polymorphism in the Scandinavian gene pool.

Most polymorphisms are not as obvious as hair or skin color. They are minuscule changes in cell proteins that may produce subtle effects on cell function. We are just beginning to discover which gene polymorphisms are important for human health, and much of that work has been led by cancer researchers trying to determine which gene polymorphisms may increase an individual's risk for cancer. In the future, dermatologists will be able to take a swab from a patient's inside cheek, and using the same cosmetic-counter gene-screen technology, make customized recommendations about sun protection or determine the best treatment choice if cancers arise.

The next step will be to extend this research to other skin concerns, such as acne, wrinkles, and aging. It is likely that some gene polymorphisms determine who has beautiful skin or who has skin that ages prematurely. Which genes could they be? We don't know yet. But that hasn't stopped a few companies from jumping way out in front and promising corrective creams that are based on personal gene analysis—unfortunately without supporting data. Such premature claims will make it harder for the real science to be accepted when it comes along.

Bottom line: Sometime soon, credible research will identify which gene polymorphisms are associated with which skin-aging processes. Armed with your own genetic profile, you'll be able to have a custom skin-care regimen designed just for you—one that will provide elements your skin is lacking and come in exactly the strength you need.

HOLISTIC MEDICINE

Holistic medicine integrates all aspects of personal health—mind, body, and spirit, working synergistically together. Spas that embrace relaxation therapy and downtime from life's regular stresses are, surprisingly, completely compatible with recent findings in molecular biology.

Holistic medicine and molecular biology both teach us that life is not a pathway but a network. We're beginning to understand the way the genetic program weaves together cells of the nervous system with those of the skin and the brain, for example, by making them responsive to a complex fabric of signaling molecules that pass between them.

This idea has completely changed the old linear way of thinking that Step A must lead to Step B, which leads to Step C. Instead, an interlaced connection with multiple paths—much like a spider web—connects Step A to Step C to Step B and back to Step A.

What fits with the new understanding of networks is new treatments that combine antioxidants that complement one another's ability to trap free radicals. Or a combination of factors that turns on the wound-healing response without a wound. You can look forward to new products with combinations of ingredients for tackling complex skin problems.

This newly understood interconnection is being closely studied by the fragrance industry. Some studies have shown that personality seems to determine a person's reaction to a particular scent. Some scents have demonstrated consistently positive effects, whether lowering heart rate, easing stress, calming anger, or improving mental concentration. The message of all these studies is simple: You smell what you are, and you are what you smell.

This knowledge is, of course, the basis for aromatherapy. Although using your sense of smell to effect medical cures is dismissed by many as nonsense, new studies may prove that scent is even more powerful than previously believed. In the next generation of skin-care products, you will choose personalized fragrances that not only address who you are, but more importantly, make you who you want to be and how you want to be seen.

Bottom line: The "soft" science of holistic medicine will combine with the "hard" science of molecular biology to form a unified network of integrated treatments for the skin. They will go way beyond what we have today into new fields like neuroscience and create science-based personal regimens combining cosmetics, training in relaxation, and aromatherapy.

IMAGING

Cameras with digital imaging give immediate, accurate pictures of your skin's appearance, and sometimes they can be devastating enough to shock even the most blasé sun worshipper into finally picking up the sunscreen.

New cameras, such as the Canfield Visia imaging system, are just beginning to make their appearance outside of specialty doctor's offices. They take digital images that can be broken down to analyze wrinkles, skin tone, pores, and sun blemishes. After a few treatments at the spa or salon, a second photo can make you into your own before-and-after study. There is nothing comparable to the gratification of actually seeing and measuring improvements to your skin to make the process and products seem worthwhile.

In the near future, you should be able to step into a kiosk in a shopping mall and get a digital photo of that spot that has been bothering you, or even a full body photo. The computer image will be transmitted hundreds of miles away to be read by a trained dermatologist, and you can get a nearly instant clean bill of health or a recommendation for a follow-up visit. That may shorten the wait times for doctors—and the convenience may even get a few men to practice a little skin-cancer prevention.

Bottom line: Cameras and computers, on a mass-market scale, will help sort out what skin-care products work and convince people to comply with their treatment program.

MULTITASKING PRODUCTS

Few women have either the time or the inclination to perform a complicated skin-care regimen at home each morning and night. One solution is to use multitasking products that can pack hydrating, calming, and collagen-building properties into one small jar.

And because we're more inclined these days to define ourselves by the stages of our lives rather than to pigeonhole ourselves according to our age, it's heartening to know that the New Skin-Care Revolution promises results based on that notion. The goal isn't better skin at age fifty, but to preserve youth and prolong healthy skin functioning no matter when you were born!

Bottom line: In the future, new products will be directed less at specific age groups or decades and more toward optimizing several skin functions at once. Good brands will be able to serve you throughout your lifetime.

NUTRITIONAL COSMETICS

Although there have been long-term studies proving that eating chocolate and French fries does not cause acne, we still don't yet have a precise understanding about which foods improve skin. That hasn't stopped some physicians and dermatologists from insisting, however, that their special diets are an integral component of their skin-care regimens. Never mind that there isn't any clinical testing or very much scientific evidence to support them!

Eating a balanced diet with fresh vegetables is now a well-established road to healthy skin. Several major cosmetic and consumer-products companies are gearing up their research to find food supplements, or nutricosmetics, that truly benefit skin. Imedeen, a Danish skin-care supplement from Farrosan Pharmaceuticals, and Innéov, a skin care and hair care supplement from L'Oréal and Nestlé, are currently available. Intelligent Nutrients from Horst Rechelbacher, the founder of Aveda, has just launched a line combining nutraceutical foods with anti-aging facial care. Expect to see many new nutritional supplements sold at the cosmetic counter in the coming years.

Before rushing out to buy nutricosmetics, though, don't forget that the first place a food supplement goes is into your stomach, which is loaded with strong acid and enzymes to digest protein and dissolve fats. Whatever remains then goes into the intestines, where the cells lining the surface secrete more degrading enzymes and then carefully pick and choose among the digested nutrients to find the right ones to be absorbed into the bloodstream. The next stop for those nutrients is a pass through the liver, which specializes in detoxifying foreign compounds.

The fact is few compounds that go into the mouth end up in the bloodstream unchanged. Complex molecules that might have anti-inflammatory or energy-boosting effects in the laboratory must survive your digestive and detoxifying systems before they can have any benefit on your skin. Hopefully, upcoming products will be able to circumvent your digestive juices and filtering by the liver to really deliver effective nutrients where they're needed.

Bottom line: Continuing research will identify nutritional supplements that actually do have benefits for the skin when they are taken orally.

SPF REACHES THE END OF THE ROAD

We have hit the wall with sunscreen. It's not that good sunscreens can't be made—it's that we can't seem to use them properly, or use enough of them to give us the SPF we think we're getting on a daily basis. On a larger scale, it's virtually impossible to change behavior so that the majority of consumers will regularly apply even a *little* dab of sunscreen in

Sunscreens of the Future

The next wave of sunscreens will have a new rating that will appear next to the SPF rating on the product label, called the IPF (immune protection factor).

IPF can be useful in a new way, as studies that test the ability of a sunscreen to protect against sunburn don't necessarily predict how much it will protect against immune suppression. In fact, sun exposure that doesn't cause sunburn can still potently inhibit natural immunity. An IPF will be able to measure how much more sun can be tolerated while using the product without getting immune suppression. Some scientists also think this is a more accurate measure of how much you're being protected from photoaging.

the right way. And even when people don't get sunburned, we now know that even a little sun is damaging their skin and their immune system. People should still use sunscreens, no doubt about it, but new approaches in protecting against sun damage and photoaging are needed if we are going to make any progress.

The ultimate goal is clear: To have effective sun protection we need to go beyond our dependence on sunscreens. One solution is to incorporate into the newest moisturizers and after-sun products enzymes that improve natural DNA repair, as well as effective combinations of antioxidants. The other solution is to follow Australia's lead and shift emphasis in the public message to more UV protective clothing, hats, and shading. Outdoor venues, like parks and sports stadiums, will likely be designed with more sun protection in mind.

STAY TUNED . . .

The next wave of the New Skin-Care Revolution is just starting to build. The more we decode the secrets of the genes—allowing us to repair and redirect our own DNA—the more science will be able to fine-tune a program for perfect skin that will last decades longer than ever before.

PART IV

REGIMENS AND RECOMMENDATIONS

■   ■   ■

THIRTEEN

Daily Regimens

A good skin-care routine isn't measured by how many products are used or how many steps are in the program. In fact, as you know by now, quite the opposite is true. All you really need are one or two comprehensive products as well as a sunscreen in the morning and a cleanser and one or two additional products at night. A regimen should only take you a few minutes—and you're done!

Comprehensive sun protection and DNA reprogramming and repair are integral aspects of these regimens. The only exception is if you have a specific skin condition, such as adult acne, hyperpigmentation, vitiligo, atopic dermatitis, or rosacea and need ongoing treatment, in which case you need to develop a program with your physician.

For more information about each step, refer to specific chapters earlier in the book.

BASIC REGIMENS

A good regimen will do the following:

1. **Cleanse**—Carefully cleanse the skin without accelerating the loss of necessary lipids (skin oils).

2. **Moisturize**—Keep the skin hydrated and provide a barrier against the elements with active ingredients.

3. Reprogram DNA—Reset the aging clock with a DNA repair enhancer along with antioxidants, which will keep skin cells functioning, reprogram the skin's lower layers to build collagen, and stimulate circulation, all to prevent and reverse wrinkles.

4. Provide Sun Protection—Minimize sun exposure and use sunscreen frequently to slow down accumulated sun damage that causes photoaged skin.

5. Brighten Skin Tone—Use a combination of a brightener, a retinol, and an exfoliator to even out skin tone. This is an optional step that need not be done all the time. If you do this step, stick to twice daily for brighteners, once daily for retinol and exfoliators, and continue until you achieve the desired results.

When you do use brighteners, retinol, and AHA/PHA products, always apply sunscreen before going out.

MORNING REGIMEN

The following are the key steps. A good multitasking product will combine more than one of these steps, so you may need to use only two products in your morning routine.

1. Cleanse your skin, gently. Use warm water alone if possible.

2. Moisturize with a multitasking product. An optimal moisturizer will include vitamins C and E to build the collagen layers, an ingredient like ursolic acid to strengthen the top barrier layer, and a calming ingredient to reduce inflammation.

3. Reprogram DNA and encourage DNA repair and recovery with key nutrients.

4. Perform optional steps for special needs, such as brightening or increasing microcirculation for dark under-eye circles.

5. Protect with sunscreen with an SPF of at least 15. Use a higher SPF if you have fair skin or a history of sun-related problems.

A few tips

▪ Use the mildest cleanser to avoid stripping the skin of much-needed lipids. Soaping your face in the shower counts as cleansing, too (but don't use body soap!).

▪ For dry skin, wash with lukewarm water in the morning and save the cleansing step for the evening, to remove makeup. Use a mild soap or nonsoap cleansers and warm but not hot water. Keep it simple with no additives—it's going to be washed away immediately.

▪ Skip the toner. It can unnecessarily dry your skin. Its effects fade in a few minutes, and it works *against* the deep penetration needed for effective moisturization. If you do have excessively oily skin and an astringent truly is needed, make sure it has alcohol or witch hazel to do the job.

▪ Never leave the house without sunscreen on!

EVENING REGIMEN

1. Cleanse your skin thoroughly to remove makeup and excess oil.

2. Moisturize with a multitasking product. An optimal moisturizer will contain vitamins C and E and encourage DNA reprogramming and repair.

3. Optional steps for special needs: For example, use a microcirculation cream if you have dark under-eye circles. Continue the brightening treatment. Alternate exfoliation and retinol treatments. Restore vitamins and antioxidants afterward with a post-peel product if they are not in your moisturizer already.

    Use an AHA/PHA exfoliation cream nightly for six weeks.

    Then use a retinol or retinoic acid (prescription) cream for
        six weeks.

    Repeat the cycle, using each product for six weeks.

A few tips

■ Cleanse only to remove makeup, but no more. Alternatives to soap are creamy or foaming cleansers. Especially effective are cleansing cloths that take off the makeup without soaking the oils out of your skin with detergent.

■ Rotate six weeks of exfoliation with six weeks of retinol—but this is a two-step process. You must restore the nutrients depleted by these treatments with a product that contains antioxidants, especially vitamins C and E.

■ Nighttime is the best time for remedial moisturization and to address skin problems. This way, the product stays on your face while you rest, is not covered by makeup, and is less likely to be wiped, rubbed, scratched, or kissed off. For those under forty, this usually means that all you'll need is a thin layer of your favorite morning moisturizer and then off to bed. Those over forty should use anti-aging moisturizers with DNA repair, circulation stimulators, or collagen building retinols. Special attention should be paid to moisturizing areas around the eyes and lips, which have less natural sebum and get dry more easily.

■ Use a lightening product if you like, but start slow to avoid irritation.

Sample Regimens

This chart will help you decide on products for a basic daily regimen. Feel free to pick and choose products that you like and customize to meet your own special needs.

Remember these points:

■ You can use the same cleanser at night as in the morning if it is able to remove makeup or you don't use any.

■ You can choose a moisturizer and a DNA repair/sunscreen product, or you can choose a moisturizer/DNA repair product and your favorite sunscreen, or you can choose three separate products: a moisturizer, a DNA repair product, and a sunscreen. It's completely up to you.

■ You can use the same moisturizer in the morning as at night.

■ Brighteners need to be used twice daily for six to eight weeks to see results.

	Morning	Evening
1. Cleanse	Dove Sensitive Skin Beauty Bar	Neutrogena Make-up Remover Cleansing Towelettes
	Cetaphil Gentle Daily Cleanser	Eau Thermale Avène Emollient Cleansing Gel with Cold Cream
	Coria CeraVe Hydrating Cleanser	
	Estée Lauder Perfectly Clean Foaming Cleanser	
2. Moisturize	Remergent Barrier Repair Formula	Repeat at night
	SkinCeuticals C E Ferulic	Repeat at night
	Cellex-C Advanced-C Serum	Repeat at night
	Remergent Antioxidant Refoliator Post-Peel Balm	Repeat at night
	Laboratoire Remède Post Peel Skin Calming Balm	Repeat at night
3. Reprogram DNA	Remergent DNA Repair Formula (moisture plus DNA repair)	Repeat at night
	Clinique Advanced Stop Signs (moisture plus DNA repair)	Repeat at night
	Amway Artistry Time Defiance Intensive Repair Serum	Repeat at night
	Estée Lauder Re-Nutriv Ultimate Lifting Creme	Repeat at night

4. Protect from sun and repair DNA	Remergent A.M. Moisture SPF 15	Not applicable
	Mary Kay TimeWise Day Solution Sunscreen SPF 25	Not applicable
Protect from sun	La Roche–Posay Anthelios XL Lait SPF 60	Not applicable
	Shiseido Ultimate Sun Protection Lotion SPF 55	Not applicable
5. Optional treatments		
Exfoliate	Not applicable	NeoStrata Exuviance Rejuvenating Complex Anti-Aging (12 percent polyhydroxy acids)
	Not applicable	GlyDerm Cream Plus 10% (10 percent glycolic acid)
Retinol—alternate with exfoliation	Not applicable	RoC Retinol Correxion Deep Wrinkle Daily Moisturizer
	Not applicable	L'Oréal Advanced RevitaLift Complete (with vitamin A)
	Not applicable	MD Formulations Vit-A-Plus
Brighten—as needed	Remergent Clarifying Concentrate[2]	Repeat at night
	Skin Effects by Dr. Jeffrey Dover Advanced Brightening Complex	Repeat at night
	Peter Thomas Roth Potent Botanical Skin Brightening Gel Complex	Repeat at night
Correct dark under-eye circles	Remergent Microcirculation Therapy	Repeat at night
	Dermal-K Clarifying Cream	Repeat at night

REGIMEN FOR CHILDREN

Children have only one skin-care need beyond cleansing: sun protection.

Sunscreen can be used on babies six months and older. Start with gentle formulas designed for sensitive young skin. Always use sunscreen on faces and exposed skin during extended periods outdoors, and reapply often.

Many kids hate having sunscreen put on, but that's not any excuse! Use a spray on your squirmiest child and reapply it often as it's not as strong as a cream. And be sure to protect infants with hats and clothing and seek out shady areas for them. They're not old enough to do it for themselves!

It is next to impossible to convince preteen children—and a great many teens, of course—to use sunscreen regularly. Lecturing them about what will happen to their skin when they grow up is all but pointless. Try another tack and buy them hats and sunglasses like those worn by their favorite idols. A baseball hat is better than nothing on a surly tween!

Remember this crucial point: DNA damage inflicted at a young age that remains unrepaired has far more years to grow into wrinkled and spot-riddled skin than the same damage sustained later in life.

REGIMEN FOR TEENAGERS WITH ACNE

For many of us, the first personal encounter we have with skin gone wrong is adolescent acne. This condition is caused by tiny inflamed sebaceous glands that become stuffed up with sebum and festering with the *P. acnes* bacteria. This is caused by the massive surge of hormonal changes, especially rising levels of those pesky androgens (male hormones, which affect women as well). Unfortunately, a massive surge in oil production means that there's more oil to clog the pores. It tenaciously binds with cell debris, and then bacteria swoop in for a meal and start to grow. Soon there's an open comedo, or blackhead, and it often progresses to become an inflamed pimple that can drive teens to despair.

Sebaceous glands are concentrated around the face, head, neck and shoulders. They start working just prior to birth, when androgens secreted by the mother and passed to the baby send signals to pump out sebum and other waxy oils that form vernix, a coating that protects the baby's skin during the birth process. Sebum production remains high in babies in their first few weeks, which is why some newborns have little pimples. The glands then tone down and remain largely dormant until puberty. And then all hell breaks loose.

Some adults also find that acne flares up when least expected (or wanted). This, too, is a result of fluctuating hormone levels. Women approaching menopause, when the feminizing hormones are declining and the male androgens remain steady, can be devastated by the appearance of breakouts. A visit to the dermatologist is usually recommended for any adult suffering from acne. Products directed at oilier teenaged skin can be much too harsh and drying for adults.

Step 1. Wash twice a day with salicylic acid

Wash no more than twice a day to remove excess sebum and bacteria. Try convincing teens of that, though. They're convinced that dirty faces cause acne. Well, they don't. (Nor do French fries or chocolate.) Hormones cause acne.

The best brands of acne washes contain a strong detergent, like sodium laureth sulfate, combined with 2 percent salicylic acid. The salicylic acid dissolves the oils and microscopic flakes of the upper skin layer that can get stuck in pores and worsen blackheads, so that these waste products can be washed away in a complete rinse.

RECOMMENDED SALICYCLIC ACID ACNE WASHES

- Bioré Pore Perfect Warming Anti-Blackhead Cream Cleanser
- Clearasil Acne Gel Cleanser
- Dermaclear All-in-One Formula

- Nature's Gate Corrective Cleansing Treatment (for the body)
- Neutrogena Oil-Free Acne Wash
- pHisoderm 4-Way Daily Acne Cleanser

Step 2. Apply benzoyl peroxide

After washing, you'll need to apply benzoyl peroxide, which unclogs pores and inhibits the growth of the *P. acnes* bacteria. Benzoyl peroxide products come as either creams or gels, and clinical studies have found that the 2.5 percent strength is about as effective as the 5 or 10 percent strength and is far less irritating.

Start out using benzoyl peroxide every other night and then build up to once or twice a day, because it still can be irritating over the long haul. It may take four to six weeks to see any improvement, so be patient.

For some, benzoyl peroxide may still be too irritating or may not seem to have much of an effect on the acne itself, so try exfoliating with some of the techniques listed in chapter 10, including the use of AHAs, BHAs such as salicylic acid, microdermabrasion, or laser treatments. Ask your dermatologist which might be best for you.

RECOMMENDED BENZOYL PEROXIDE PRODUCTS

- Jan Marini Benzoyl Peroxide Wash 2.5%
- Neutrogena On-the-Spot Acne Treatment Vanishing Formula
- Proactiv Solution (The second step of their three-step program, Revitalizing Toner, contains witch hazel for drying. For some this can be a serious irritant, especially when combined with so many other strong drying and irritating agents.)
- Solvére Acne Clearing Gel

TREATING ACNE WITH PRESCRIPTION DRUGS

If an OTC regimen with the salicylic acid/benzoyl peroxide combination doesn't work after several months of use, it's time for a consultation with a dermatologist experienced in treating acne.

Topical Antibiotics

The first try is usually a topical antibiotic, such as erythromycin or clindamycin. Although they work for about half of those who try them, getting teens to use them consistently is a real problem. A clindamycin phosphate gel (such as Clindagel) might help, as it can be applied simply by rubbing it on gently with fingers once a day.

Retinoic Acid

The most effective anti-acne drugs are derived from retinoic acid, the active form of vitamin A. Earlier versions worked well on acne but were often quite irritating. In the 1990s, retinoic acid was re-engineered to produce two new anti-acne drugs, adapalene and tazarotene, which shut down sebum secretion and prevent the *P. acnes* bacteria from taking over the pores. A bonus is that adapalene and tazarotene can also be used, like Retin-A, to reduce wrinkles and rejuvenate skin. But they may cause birth defects and must never be used by women who are pregnant.

Isotretinoin

The most potent anti-acne drug is the oral form of retinoic acid called isotretinoin. Its brand name is Accutane.

Accutane is very effective for severe, cystic acne; but it often has side effects, such as dry skin, muscle aches, bone spurs, and increased sun sensitivity. It can also cause birth defects, so beginning in 2006, everyone who takes Accutane, male or female, must enroll in iPledge, a national registry mandated by the FDA. Teenaged girls or adult women must submit pregnancy tests before Accutane is dispensed.

Further controversy has erupted over whether Accutane increases the risk of suicide. But a close review of the data finds little to support this link. Discuss any concerns with your dermatologist.

INGREDIENTS TO AVOID IF YOU HAVE ACNE

Most girls begin to experiment with cosmetics and makeup when they hit the teen years, but this can be a nightmare for anyone with a bad case of acne. Makeup often contains ingredients that are comedogenic, meaning that they increase the risk of clogging up sebaceous glands and pores. And the more acne there is, the more desperate a teen can be to cover it up, exacerbating an already inflamed face with more oil and irritants.

Anyone with acne should read labels carefully and avoid using products with these ingredients:

Butyl stearate
Lanolin
Lauryl alcohol
Oleic acid
Vegetable butters or oils
Waxes

MEN AND SKIN CARE

From talking to most men about skin care, you would think we were a different species! Oh, sure, a lot more men in their twenties and thirties have started using cleansers and moisturizers, and the men's skin-care industry is growing twice as fast as women's, but the fact remains that men's cosmetics are still a very small fraction of the market. Men think that advertisements depicting men's skin problems are "fearmongering." Of course, some of this bluster is cloaking the macho attitude that skin care and cosmetics are effeminate and that concern about looks might appear as vanity. Plus they know that our society still tells us that a man with wrinkles is distinguished but a woman with wrinkles is just plain old.

So most men claim they don't have skin problems, aside from razor bumps or the occasional sunburn. This was proven to me when our lab gathered two focus groups to discuss the types of skin-care products they were likely to use. The first group was composed of ten men from their mid-thirties to mid-forties, who did purchase skin-care products and go to spas regularly. Despite their obvious concern for their appearance, when they were advised that their skin had suffered sun damage and that products were available to help them stave off signs of aging, their nearly universal response was complete denial. These men said that so long as they felt good, they would look good. Any evidence to the contrary, they declared, was a hoax designed to coerce them into buying skin-care products they did not need and that, by the way, never really worked anyway.

The second group was composed of ten cosmetics-conscious women in the same age range. They understood the skin-damage and product-solution issues immediately and held a lively discussion of which cosmetics they used and why. And despite the great range of education and careers in the room, they were in agreement that nothing guided them in their choices better than trial and error. Some frankly admitted that they would try anything to rejuvenate their skin.

It's too bad men don't feel the same way, as they have a few special concerns due to more active sebaceous glands, androgens, and coarse facial hair. On the one hand, male hormones stimulate more sebum production, so men's skin tends to be less dry than women's. On the other hand, a man without a beard may shave more than twenty thousand times during his lifetime—and each shave is tantamount to a mini-exfoliation.

Which means men need a moisturizer—whether they think they do or not!—particularly one that also replenishes depleted antioxidants and has an anti-irritant effect to calm shaved skin. A good moisturizer for men should contain aloe or chamomile, but preferably licorice extract or evodia, as well as those essential vitamins A, B_3, C, and E. It should be used not just on the beard area but massaged gently into the temples and the area around the eyes (but not too close). Save a little for the front and back of the neck, the ears (especially on top), and the skin above the collarbone.

Without moisturization, a man's skin can end up as tough as leather. And sun exposure will further toughen that leather into a creased mess. Men who refuse to use sunscreen on its own should at least try to use a daily moisturizer with an SPF of at least 15.

What men don't need are alcohol-laden aftershaves, as they're unnecessarily drying. The brace of the aftershave splash and the cool sensation brought on by the evaporation can be as addictive as toners are for many women, so for men used to dabbing it on, smoothing on a lotion or a cream instead may seem unsettling. But if they stick with it, the aftershave will soon be forgotten. (A scented aftershave can also be replaced with a dab or spray of a favorite cologne—but don't forget that the concentration of fragrance in cologne is much higher than in an aftershave, so be sparing in its use.)

The one skin-care issue that motivates men more than any other is baldness. Many men spend their adult years on a never-ending quest for a magical hair-restoration elixir. Unfortunately, there are few new treatments. The promise of minoxidil, which was discovered during research on heart disease to stimulate blood flow to the hair follicle, has fallen short for many, but not all, men. In fact the clinical studies supporting it measured the improvement by the number of new individual hairs per square inch, not by new patches covering square inches of baldness. For men just starting to lose their hair, the prescription drug Propecia blocks the metabolism of a male hormone that contributes to hair loss. This might slow down the balding process, but it can't significantly reverse it. And for men who are already bald, there are no scientifically supported products available (despite countless claims to the contrary) that can regrow a head of hair.

The most promising line of research treats baldness as an autoimmune disease in which the immune system attacks and shuts down hair follicles. Safe but effective topical immune suppressants may someday be able to stop the assault and permit hair to regrow.

Bald men especially are prone to sun damage, precancers, and cancers on their heads. But all men in general need to practice safe sun, not only for their looks, but for their health. They need sunscreen as much as women do!

Fortunately, a growing number of men are using a new generation of medically oriented skin-care lines such as DDF, Murad, Remergent, and SkinCeuticals, which tend to be non–gender specific. They might also like skin-care lines that are either gender neutral, such as Malin+Goetz or Dr. Brandt, or lines designed specifically for men, such as Anthony Logistics for Men, Jack Black, and Zirh.

Or, if they're really smart, they'll start borrowing the same products used by the women in their lives!

Bottom line: Men need skin-care products as much as women do, no matter how much they deny it. At the top of the list are moisturizing and SPF items, and they can put aside the aftershave. Cosmetic treatments for baldness are full of unproven hype, so stick to the proven prescription and OTC drugs, such as minoxidil or Propecia.

RECOMMENDED PRODUCTS FOR MEN

Note: Although the best men's products are not as expensive as women's, they are not as easily found in drugstores and mass-market shops.

* Anthony Logistics for Men All Purpose Facial Moisturizer
* Anthony Logistics for Men Pre-Shave Oil
* Clinique Skin Supplies for Men Face Scrub
* Dr. Brandt "A" Cream
* Jack Black Double-Duty Face Moisturizer SPF 20
* Lab Series Skincare for Men Razor Burn Relief Ultra
* Malin+Goetz Replenishing Face Serum
* Malin+Goetz Vitamin E Face Moisturizer
* Remergent Barrier Repair Formula
* The Art of Shaving After-Shave Gel
* The Art of Shaving Moisturizer
* Zirh Soothe Post-Shave Solution

■   ■   ■

FOURTEEN

The Master Product List

This chapter contains all the products recommended in this book organized by steps in my simplified regimen. This is designed to help you choose wisely at the store or on the Internet. Don't hesitate to take it with you to the store or have it next to the computer when you order products online.

Note: The products in this list are all preceded by a symbol:

✹ denotes luxury products
• denotes drugstore products

Luxury products (✹) are those that are high priced (usually more than forty dollars a bottle) and are found at department store cosmetic counters, specialty stores, or on the Internet. They usually have limited distribution.

Drugstore products (•) are those that are more moderately priced (usually less than forty dollars a bottle) and are widely found in chain drugstores, supermarkets, mass-market stores like Wal-Mart and Target, television shopping shows, and from personal sales companies like Amway, Avon, and Mary Kay.

The ways cosmetic products are sold are changing rapidly, and there are no hard and fast rules about where products may be found. What follows is only a guideline to help locate the products you want.

STEP 1: CLEANSING

MORNING CLEANSERS—MILD

Bar Cleansers

- Basis Sensitive Skin Bar
- Dove Sensitive Skin Beauty Bar
- Purpose Gentle Cleansing Bar

Liquid Cleansers

- Bioré Foaming Liquid Cleanser
- Cetaphil Gentle Daily Cleanser
- Dove Sensitive Skin Foaming Facial Cleanser
- ❀ Estée Lauder Perfectly Clean Foaming Cleanser
- ❀ Garden Botanika Skin Renewing Gentle Foaming Cleanser
- Olay Foaming Face Wash
- ❀ Shiseido Pureness Cleansing Gel

EVENING CLEANSERS—SIMPLE CLEANSING

Cleansing Cloths

- Dove Facial Cleansing Cloths
- Neutrogena Make-up Remover Cleansing Towlettes
- Olay Daily Facials Cleansing Cloths

Liquid Cleansers

- Aveeno Clear Complexion Foaming Cleanser
- Eau Thermale Avéne Emollient Cleansing Gel with Cold Cream
- ❀ Clarins Cleansing Milk
- ❀ Clinique Wash-Away Gel Cleanser
- ❀ Dr. Hauschka Cleansing Milk
- ❀ Givenchy Clean It Tender Creamy Cleansing Foam
- Neutrogena Deep Clean Facial Cleanser
- ❀ Peter Thomas Roth Chamomile Cleansing Lotion
- ❀ T. Leclerc Gentle Cleansing Milk

Cleansers with Added Ingredients

Not recommended unless you are willing to pay extra for unnecessary ingredients with a nice feel.

- ✹ DERMAdoctor Wrinkle Revenge Antioxidant Enhanced Glycolic Acid Facial Cleanser
- ✹ Exuviance Purifying Cleansing Gel
- ✹ Joey New York Calm and Correct Gentle Soothing Cleanser
- Mary Kay TimeWise 3-in-1 Cleanser
- ✹ M.D. Forté Facial Lotion I (15 percent glycolic acid)
- ✹ Murad AHA/BHA Exfoliating Cleanser

STEPS 2 AND 3:
MOISTURIZE AND REPROGRAM DNA

OLDER GENERATION MOISTURIZERS

Facial Use—With Added Sunscreen

- Amway Artistry Time Defiance Day Protect Crème SPF 15
- Dove Deep Moisture Facial Lotion For Dry Skin with SPF 15
- ✹ Estée Lauder DayWear Plus SPF 30
- L'Oréal Advanced RevitaLift Cream or Lotion SPF 15
- L'Oréal Dermo-Expertise Futur*e Moisture+a Daily Dose of Pure Vitamin E, SPF 15
- Mary Kay TimeWise Age-Fighting Moisturizer Sunscreen SPF 15
- Neutrogena Healthy Skin Face Lotion SPF 15
- Olay Complete All Day Moisture Lotion SPF 15
- Olay Total Effects 7X Visible Anti-Aging Vitamin Complex with UV Protection
- Pond's Mend & Defend Intensive Protection SPF 15

Facial Use—Without Sunscreen

- Clean & Clear Oil-Free Dual Action Moisturizer
- ✹ Clinique Dramatically Different Moisturizing Lotion
- ✹ H_2O Plus Face Oasis Hydrating Treatment

- Neutrogena Advanced Solutions Skin Transforming Complex Nightly Renewal Cream

Body Use
- Curél Ultra Healing Intensive Moisture Lotion
- Eucerin Aquaphor
- Eucerin Calming Cream
- Jergens Age Defying Lotion Multi-Vitamin Moisturizer
- Lubriderm Daily Moisture
- Lubriderm Sensitive Moisture
- Mary Kay TimeWise Cellu-Shape Daytime Body Moisturizer
- Neutrogena Norwegian Formula Body Moisturizer
- ❀ Origins A Perfect World Highly Hydrating Body Lotion
- Vaseline Intensive Care Firming Radiance Age-Defying Lotion
- Vaseline Intensive Care Healthy Body Complexion Nourishing Body Lotion

NEW SKIN-CARE REVOLUTION MOISTURIZERS

A good moisturizer can do a lot more than keep your skin hydrated. Look for multitasking moisturizers that contain the following: humectant base that is gentle and easy to apply; botanicals to build the outer barrier and strengthen collagen; ingredients that stimulate DNA repair; agents that calm skin and reduce irritation. For those with few skin-care issues, your program can have the same moisturizer morning and night. For those with problems to address, consider a moisturizer tackling some in the morning and a different one directed to other problems at night.

Calming
- Eucerin Redness Relief Soothing Night Creme
- ❀ Laboratoire Remède Post Peel Skin Calming Balm
- ❀ Lindi Soothing Balm
- ❀ Oils of Aloha Kukui Essential AfterSun Lotion
- ❀ Remergent Barrier Repair Formula

Collagen Builders
* ❃ Cellex-C Advanced-C Serum
* ❃ MD Formulations Vit-A-Plus
* ❃ Remergent Microcirculation Therapy
* • RoC Retinol Correxion Deep Wrinkle Daily Moisturizer
* ❃ SkinCeuticals C E Ferulic

Dark Under-Eye Circles—Vitamin K and Diols
* ❃ Dermal-K Clarifying Cream
* ❃ Dermalogics Eyederma
* ❃ Donell Skin Care K-Derm Gel or Cream (formerly known as Super-Skin)
* ❃ Jason Vitamin K Crème Plus
* ❃ Remergent Microcirculation Therapy
* ❃ Skin Amnesty Regenerating Eye Cream

DNA Repair
* • Amway Artistry line
* • Avon beComing Un-Flawed Damage Recovery Complex
* ❃ Clinique Advanced Stop Signs
* ❃ Estée Lauder Re-Nutriv Ultimate Lifting Creme
* • Mary Kay TimeWise Day Solution Sunscreen SPF 25
* ❃ Neways NightScience
* ❃ Neways Rebound After Sun Lotion
* ❃ Nu Skin 180° UV Block Hydrator SPF 18
* • Olay Definity Correcting Protective Lotion SPF 15
* ❃ Origins Make A Difference
* ❃ Remergent A.M. Moisturizer SPF 15
* ❃ Remergent DNA Repair Formula
* ❃ Remergent High Intensity SPF 30

Isoflavones (Plant Estrogens)—Antioxidants and Hydrating
* • Aveeno Positively Radiant Daily Moisturizer SPF 15
* ❃ DDF Silky C (with retinol, soy, and lutein)

* Earth Therapeutics Clari-T First Aid Kit
* KaplanMD Phytogenic Triactive Complex Perfecting Serum
* Lamas Botanicals Soy Nourishing Moisturizer
* Reviva Labs Soy Intensive Rejuvenating Serum
* SoySoft Daily Moisturizing Body Lotion

B Vitamins (Niacinamide) — Strengthens Barrier and Brightens

* Aveeno Active Naturals Positively Radiant Anti-Wrinkle Cream
* H_2O Plus Face Oasis Hydrating Treatment
* Lumene Vitamin+ Vita-Nectar Vitalizing Day Cream SPF 15
* Olay Regenerist Continuous Night Recovery Moisturizing Treatment
* Olay Total Effects 7X Visible Anti-Aging Vitamin Complex

Ursolic Acid — Strengthens Barrier

* Avon Anew Alternative Intensive Age Treatment SPF 25 Day
* Charmzone Wrinklear Cream
* Natura Bissé Diamond Body Cream
* Pola Day+Day Vitax Wrinkle Shot
* Remergent Barrier Repair Formula
* Ren Frankincense and *Boswellia Serrata* Revitalising Repair Cream
* Sisley Global Anti-Age Cream

Immune Enhancers with Aloe

* Clinique After-Sun Balm with Aloe
* Herbalife Herbal Aloe Hand Cream
* Magic of Aloe Nourishing Moisture Lotion
* Optima Organic Aloe Vera Lotion
* Skin MD Natural Dry Skin Care Treatment Shielding Lotion

Immune Enhancers with Tamarind

* Breathe Delight Multi-Vitamin Hand Cream
* Harmony of Thai Yoghurt Tamarind Body Lotion
* Molton Brown Skinboost 24hr Moisture Mist

STEP 4: SUN PROTECTION

Find broad-spectrum sunscreens with at least an SPF 15 for use every day as well as a sunscreen with an SPF 30 or higher when you expect to spend more time in the sun. The best sunscreen will also contain vitamins C and E and DNA repair ingredients (if these are not already in your moisturizer).

No one type of sunscreen is suitable for everyone. Find one you like by trying those with chemical sunscreens, then physical sunscreens. If you can get your hands on sunscreens with the latest ingredients from Europe (Mexoryl or Tinosorb), try them first.

Sunscreens are the last product to apply every morning. Apply as much as you feel comfortable putting on and then some. Make their use as much a part of your daily routine as brushing your teeth.

Sunscreens with Chemical Sunscreens (Avobenzone plus Octisalate or Octylcrylene)

- Coppertone Endless Summer Ultrasheer Sunscreen SPF 15
- DERMAdoctor Body Guard Exquisitely Light SPF 30
- Estée Lauder Multi-Protection Sun Lotion for Body SPF 30
- Hawaiian Tropic Ozone Sport Sunblock SPF 60+
- Kiehl's Vital Sun Protection All-Sport Year-Round Face & Body Spray SPF 25
- La Roche–Posay Biomedic Facial Shield SPF 30
- Neutrogena Age Shield Sunblock with Helioplex SPF 45
- PCA Skin for Men Total Defense Calming Hydrator SPF 25
- Remergent A.M. Moisture SPF 15 Sunscreen
- RoC Age Diminishing Daily Moisturizer SPF 15

Sunscreens with Physical Sunscreens (Titanium Dioxide and/or Zinc Oxide plus Octinoxate)

- Blue Lizard Australian Suncream—Regular SPF 30+
- Cellex-C Sun Care SPF 30+
- Eucerin Dry Skin Therapy Facial Moisturizing Lotion SPF 25
- M.D. Forté Environmental Protection Cream SPF 30

- ✿ Remergent High Intensity SPF 30 Sunscreen
- ✿ Shiseido Ultimate Sun Protection Lotion SPF 55
- ✿ SunSmart Maximum Protection SPF 30 Lotion

Sunscreens with Mexoryl

- • La Roche–Posay Anthelios SX Daily Moisturizing Cream SPF 15
- ✿ La Roche–Posay Anthelios XL Lait SPF 60
- • Lancôme UV Expert SPF 20
- ✿ L'Oréal Solar Expertise 50+

Sunscreens with Tinosorb

- ✿ Bioderma Spot SPF 100
- ✿ Ducray Gel-Crème SPF 15, 30 or 50+

Spray Sunscreens

- ✿ Clinique Sun-Care Body Spray SPF 30
- • Coppertone Continuous Spray SPF 30
- ✿ Kiehl's Vital Sun Protection All-Sport Year-Round Face & Body Spray SPF 25
- • Neutrogena Fresh Cooling Body Mist Sunblock SPF 30
- • Neutrogena Healthy Defense Oil-Free Sunblock Spray SPF 30
- ✿ Vichy Capital Soleil Spray SPF 30 product line

STEP 5: EXTRA STEPS

ANTIOXIDANTS

Vitamins A, C, and E are important to maintain optimal skin health. Don't substitute other antioxidants for these vitamins. Ergothioneine is also a natural component of the skin's antioxidant defense and needs to be maintained at optimum levels. Serious scientists admit that for other kinds of antioxidants, especially plant antioxidants, there is very little evidence that applying them will provide any real benefit. When you apply natural antioxidant products, the goal is to restore and maintain natural levels; megadoses aren't any more effective and may even damage the skin. Don't use products with only one antioxidant, as they need to work in teams in order to be effective.

DNA Repair Antioxidants
* Estée Lauder Re-Nutriv Ultimate Lifting Serum
* Remergent Antioxidant Refoliator
* Remergent DNA Repair Formula

Ergothioneine with Vitamin C
* Cellex-C Advanced-C Neck Firming Cream
* Cellex-C Advanced-C Serum
* Cellex-C Advanced-C Skin Tightening Cream
* Remergent Antioxidant Refoliator
* Remergent Barrier Repair Formula
* Remergent Clarifying Concentrate

Ergothioneine without Vitamin C
* Botáge IDB Advanced Facial Anti-Oxidant Formula
* Dior No-Age Essentiel Progress Age-Defense Refining Creme
* Elizabeth Arden Ceramide Eye Wish
* Kinerase Hydrating Antioxidant Mist
* Kinerase Lip Treatment
* Neways NightScience
* Neways Rebound
* Neways Retention Plus
* Neways Skin Enhancer
* Zenyaku Kogyo Gelée Rich Pure Injuvenate Essence

Retinol
* EmerginC Multi-Vitamin and Retinol Serum
* MD Formulations Vit-A-Plus line
• Neutrogena Healthy Skin Anti-Wrinkle Cream
* Replenix Retinol Smoothing Serum 10X
• RoC Retinol Correxion Deep Wrinkle Daily Moisturizer

Sunscreens

- Lancôme Bienfait Multi-Vital SPF 30 Sunscreen
- Murasun Daily Sunblock with Antioxidants SPF 15
- Pharmaskincare Cover Mild SPF 15 Antioxidant

Vitamin Combination

- Cellex-C Advanced-C Serum
- Cosmedicine MegaDose Skin Fortifying Serum
- H_2O Plus Face Oasis Hydrating Treatment
- MDSkincare Anti-Aging Vitamin C Gel
- Olay Total Effects 7X Visible Anti-Aging Vitamin Complex with UV Protection
- Remergent Antioxidant Refoliator Post-Peel Balm
- SkinCeuticals C E Ferulic

EXFOLIATION

Exfoliation revitalizes the topmost layer of your skin, but continual exfoliation depletes that layer of important nutrients. It also increases sun sensitivity. The most effective antiwrinkle regimen alternates an AHA, BHA, or PHA exfoliant for six weeks with a retinol product for six weeks.

Don't overdo the use of exfoliants, and always follow their use with a replenishing product containing antioxidants.

AHA and PHA Exfoliants

- GlyDerm Cream Plus 10% (10 percent glycolic acid)
- M.D. Forté Lotion I (15 percent glycolic acid)
- NeoStrata Exuviance Rejuvenating Complex (12 percent polyhydroxy acids)

Postexfoliation Antioxidants

- Cellex-C Advanced-C Serum
- Remergent Antioxidant Refoliator Post-Peel Balm
- SkinCeuticals C E Ferulic
- Skin Culture Matrix Booster

LIGHTENING AND BRIGHTENING

Cosmetic brighteners work best when applied twice daily. When you use them in the morning, *always* follow with a sunscreen, or you'll undo all the benefits.

Lighteners:

Arbutin

* ❀ DHC Alpha-Arbutin White Cream
* ❀ Shiseido Whitess Intensive Skin Brightener

Ergothioneine

* ❀ Cellex-C Advanced-C Eye Firming Cream
* ❀ Remergent Clarifying Concentrate[2]
* ❀ ShiKai Adult Formula Borage Dry Skin Therapy Lotion

Hydroquinone

* Dr. Jan Adams Women of Color Skin Lightener
* Esotérica Fade Cream Regular
* ❀ Exuviance Essential Skin Lightener Gel
* ❀ Porcelana Skin Lightening Serum
* Skin Effects by Dr. Jeffrey Dover Advanced Brightening Complex

Sepiwhite

* ❀ Dr. Temt White Serum
* ❀ Elizabeth Halen Sepiwhite Lipo-Facial Cream
* ❀ Remergent Clarifying Concentrate[2]

Brighteners:

Azelaic Acid

* ❀ DDF Intensive Holistic Lightener
* ❀ Jan Marini Skin Research Factor-A Plus Mask
* ❀ Peter Thomas Roth Potent Botanical Skin Brightening Gel Complex

Kojic Acid

* GreatSkin Fruit Acid Gel with Kojic Acid 15%
* Neova Kojic Complex Gel
* Reviva Brown Spot Night Gel

Retinol

* Replenix Retinol Smoothing Serum 10X

Vitamin C

* DHC White Cream

Retinol and Vitamin C

* EmerginC Multi-Vitamin and Retinol Serum

SUNLESS TAN

Bronzing Makeup

* Bare Escentuals i.d. bareMinerals All-Over Face Color
* Estée Lauder In the Sun Shimmer Sunscreen SPF 15
* Guerlain Terracotta Fresh Bronzing Gel
* IsaDora Bronzing Powder
* Laura Mercier Bronzing Powder
* Lorac Bronzer
* Nars Bronzing Powder
* Tarte Mineral Powder Bronzer
* Vincent Longo Sole Mio Duo Bronzer

Self-Tanners

* Clarins Self Tanning Instant Gel
* Clinique Self-Sun Body Self-Tanning Mist
* Coppertone Endless Summer Sunless Tanning Lotion
* Dior Bronze Self-Tanner Natural Glow
* Estée Lauder Sun Performance Self Tan Towelettes
* Neutrogena Instant Bronze Sunless Tanner and Bronzer in One

ADDITIONAL PRODUCTS

STRESS REDUCERS

Stress has been shown to have detrimental effects on skin—effects that are visible to the naked eye and can be measured clinically. It's fair to assume than an overall reduction in stress can improve your skin's barrier function and strengthen your immune system.

While these products are not strong enough to reduce all stress, when used as part of a relaxation program, they'll help reduce symptoms and should improve your skin.

Aromatherapy

- Dead Sea Salts Relaxing Lavender Aromatherapy Bath Salt
- Jason Meditation Masque Aromatherapy
- Kaori Revitalizing Ylang Ylang Body Lotion
- Lancôme Aroma Tonic spray
- Origins Peace of Mind Cease and Destress Diffuser

ACNE

Serious acne requires medical attention from an experienced dermatologist, and none of these products are intended to treat it. But you can lessen breakouts by removing oil and targeting acne-causing bacteria with benzoyl peroxide. Salicylic acid helps dislodge cell debris from pores.

Benzoyl Peroxide Products

- Jan Marini Benzoyl Peroxide Wash 2.5%
- Neutrogena On-the-Spot Acne Treatment Vanishing Formula
- Proactive Solution (The second step of their three-step program, Revitalizing Toner, contains witch hazel for drying. For some this can be a serious irritant, especially when combined with so many other strong drying and irritating agents.)
- Solvére Acne Clearing Gel

Salicylic Acid Acne Washes

- Bioré Pore Perfect Warming Anti-Blackhead Cream Cleanser
- Clearsil Acne Gel Cleanser
- Dermaclear All-in-One Formula
- Nature's Gate Corrective Cleansing Treatment (for the body)
- Neutrogena Oil-Free Acne Wash
- pHisoderm 4-Way Daily Acne Cleanser

MEN'S SKIN CARE

Men's skin is not so very different from women's, so they don't really need special products. Of course, if you want men to stop pilfering *your* products or encourage them to take better care of their skin, you may want to consider some of these products, which are either unisex or designed for men.

RECOMMENDED PRODUCTS FOR MEN

- Anthony Logistics for Men All Purpose Facial Moisturizer
- Anthony Logistics for Men Pre-Shave Oil
- Clinique Skin Supplies for Men Face Scrub
- Dr. Brandt "A" Cream
- Jack Black Double-Duty Face Moisturizer SPF 20
- Lab Series Skincare for Men Razor Burn Relief Ultra
- Malin+Goetz Replenishing Face Serum
- Malin+Goetz Vitamin E Face Moisturizer
- Remergent Barrier Repair Formula
- The Art of Shaving After-Shave Gel
- The Art of Shaving Moisturizer
- Zirh Soothe Post-Shave Solution

NOTES

Chapter 2

1. *Q-Pharma, Inc. v Andrew Jergens Corp.,* No. C01-1312 (Western District of Washington State, Sept. 10, 2003).

Chapter 3

1. *Nicholas V. Perricone, M.D. v. Medicis Pharmaceutical Corporation* No: 05-1022, 1023 (U.S. Court of Appeals for the Federal Circuit, Dec. 20, 2005).

Chapter 9

1. *Integr Cancer Ther* 3:279, 2004.
2. *Cochrane Database System Review* 18:CD004183, 2004.
3. *JAMA* 297:842, 2007.
4. (-)-epigallocatechin-3-gallate.
5. *Br J Dermatol* 149:841, 2003.
6. *J Cosmet Dermatol* 4:11, 2005.

Chapter 10

1. *Dermatol Surg* 32:184, 2006.

BIBLIOGRAPHY

■   ■   ■

Agache, P., et al. Sebum levels during the first year of life. Br J Dermatol 103:643–49, 1980.

Aiello, A., et al. Relationship between triclosan and susceptibilities of bacteria isolated from hands in the community. Antimicrob Agents Chemother 48:2973–79, 2004.

———. Antibacterial cleaning products and drug resistance. Emerg Infect Dis 11:1565–70, 2005.

Akhavan, A., and Bershad, S. Topical acne drugs: review of clinical properties, systemic exposure, and safety. Am J Clin Dermatol 4:473–92, 2003.

Al-Attar, A., et al. Keloid pathogenesis and treatment. Plast Reconstr Surg 117:286–300, 2006.

Altermus, M., et al. Immune function in PTSD. Ann NY Acad Sci 1071:167–83, 2006.

An, K., et al. Cyclooxygenase-2 expression in murine and human nonmelanoma skin cancers. Photochem Photobiol 76:73–80, 2002.

Aramaki J., et al. Differences of skin irritation between Japanese and European women. Br J Dermatol 146:1052–56, 2002.

Arck, P. Neuroimmunology of stress: skin takes center stage. J Invest Dermatol 126:1697–1704, 2006.

Armstrong, C., and Vashon, R. Topical antimicrobial drug products for over-the-counter human use. Procter & Gamble letter to FDA, August 19, 2003.

Arndt, K., et al. Photodamage treatments. Supplement to Skin & Aging, 2004.

Autier, P., et al. Sunscreen use and intentional exposure to ultraviolet A and B radiation: a double blind randomized trial using personal dosimeters. Br J Cancer 83:1243–48, 2000.

Babcock, T., et al. Experimental studies defining omega-3 fatty acid anti-inflammatory mechanisms and abrogation of tumor-related syndromes. Nutr Clin Pract 20:62–74, 2005.

Baliga, M., and Katiyar, S. Chemoprevention of photocarcinogenesis by selected dietary botanicals. Photochem Photobio Sci 5:243–53, 2006.

Balina, L., and Graupe, K. The treatment of melasma. 20% azelaic acid versus 4% hydroquinone cream. Int J Dermatol 30:893–95, 1991.

Beer, K. Comparative evalution of the safety and efficacy of botulinum toxin type A and topical creams for treating moderate-to-severe glabellar rhytids. Dermatol Surg 32:184–92, 2006.

Beitner, H. Randomized, placebo-controlled, double blind study on the clinical efficacy of a cream containing 5% alpha-lipoic acid related to photoageing of facial skin. Br J Dermatol 149:841–49, 2003.

Berardesca, E., and Maibach, H. Ethnic skin: overview of structure and function. J Am Acad Dermatol 48:S139–42, 2003.

Berwick, M., et al. Screening for cutaneous melanoma by skin self-examination. J Natl Cancer Inst 88:17–23, 1996.

Bickers, D., and Athar, M. Oxidative stress in the pathogenesis of skin disease. J Invest Dermatol 126:2565–75, 2006.

Bikowski, J. Mechanisms of the comedolytic and anti-inflammatory properties of topical retinoids. J Drugs Dermatol 4:41–47, 2005.

Bissett, D., et al. Topical niacinamide provides skin aging appearance benefits while enhancing barrier function. Am J Clin Dermatol 32:S9–S18, 2003.

———. Niacinamide: a B vitamin that improves aging facial skin appearance. Dermatol Surg 31:860–65, 2005.

Bjelakovic, G., et al. Mortality in randomized trials of antioxidant supplements for primary and secondary prevention. JAMA 297:842–57, 2007.

Blanes-Mira, C., et al. A synthetic hexapeptide (Argireline) with antwrinkle activity. Int J Cosmet Sci 24:303–10, 2002.

Boschert, S. Cause often elusive for severe, refractory itch. Skin and Allergy News, Aug. 2006, p. 26.

Both, D., et al. Liposome-encapsulated ursolic acid increases ceramides and collagen in human skin cells. Arch Dermatol Res 293:569–75, 2002.

Brattsand, M., et al. A proteolytic cascade of kallikreins in the stratum corneum. J Invest Dermatol 124:198–203, 2005.

Breathnach, A. Melanin hyperpigmentation of skin: melasma, topical treatment with azelaic acid, and other therapies. Cutis 57:36–45, 1996.

Broccardo, M. Sauvagine: effects on thermoregulation in the rat. Pharmacol Res 22:189–96, 1990.

Brooke, R., et al. Discordance between facial wrinkling and the presence of basal cell carcinoma. Arch Dermatol 137:751–54, 2001.

Brown, D. Skin pigmentation enhancers. J Photochem Photobiol 63:148–61, 2001.

Brown, D., et al. Bicyclic monoterpene diols stimulate release of nitric oxide from skin cells, increase microcirculation and elevate skin temperature. Nitric Oxide 15:70–76, 2006.

Carlson, K., et al. Inhibition of mouse melanoma cell proliferation by corticotrophin-releasing hormone and its analogs. Anticancer Res 21:1173–79, 2001.

Chiu, V., and Weinstock, M. Incidence, mortality and the importance of early detection. The Melanoma Letter 25(1): 1–3, 2007.

Choi, E., et al. Mechanisms by which psychologic stress alters cutaneous permeability, barrier homeostasis, and stratum corneum integrity. J Invest Dermatol 124:587–95, 2005.

Colavincenzo, M., and Granstein, R. Stress and the skin: a meeting report of the Weill Cornell symposium on the science of dermatology. J Invest Dermatol 126:2560–61, 2006.

Darvin, M., et al. Effect of supplemented and topically applied antioxidant substances on human tissue. Skin Pharmacol Physiol 19:238–47, 2006.

Davidson, J., et al. Ascorbate differentially regulates elastin and collagen biosynthesis in vascular smooth muscle cells and skin fibroblasts by pretranslational mechanisms. J Biol Chem 272:345–52, 1997.

DeGroot, J. The AGE of the matrix: chemistry, consequence and cure. Cur Opin Pharmacol 4:301–5, 2004.

Dente, K. Stress affects psoriasis in most patients. Skin and Allergy News, Aug. 2006, p. 21.

Diffey, B. Climate change, ozone depletion and the impact on ultraviolet exposure of human skin. Phys Med Biol 49:R1–11, 2004.

Distante, F. Objective evaluation of the placebo effect in cosmetic treatments. IFSCC Magazine 9:203–8, 2006.

Dokka, S., et al. Dermal delivery of topically applied oligonucleotides via follicular transport in mouse skin. J Invest Dermatol 124:971–75, 2005.

Dorr, R., et al. Effects of a superpotent melanotropic peptide in combination with solar UV radiation on tanning of the skin in human volunteers. Arch Dermatol 140:827–35, 2004.

Draelos, Z. Cosmeceuticals. China: Elsevier Saunders, 2005.

———. Topical cosmeceuticals attempting to mimic injectable botulinum toxin—is it possible? Cosmet Dermatol 18:521–22, 2005.

Draelos, Z., et al. The effect of 2% niacinamide on facial sebum production. J Cosmet Laser Ther 8:96–101, 2005.

———. Site-specific product formulation, part 3: body and intertriginous skin. J Cosmet Dermatol 19:395–96, 2006.

Dreher, F., et al. Effect of topical antioxidants on UV-induced erythema formation when administered after exposure. Dermatology 198:52–55, 1999.

———. Topical melatonin in combination with vitamins E and C protects skin
from ultraviolet-induced erythema: a human study *in vivo*. Br J Deramtol
139:332–39, 1998.

Dyer, D., et al. Accumulation of Maillard reaction products in skin collagen in diabetes and aging. J Clin Invest 91:2463–69, 1993.

Eivindson, M., et al. Insulin-like growth factors (IGFs) and IGF binding proteins
in active Crohn's disease treated with omega-3 or omega-6 fatty acids and
corticosteroids. Scand J Gastroenterol 40:1214–21, 2005.

Elson, M. Method of treating blood vessel disorders of the skin using vitamin K.
US Patent 5,510,391, issued Apr. 23, 1996.

Epstein, H. Kinerase: the science behind the technology. SkinMed, Nov/Dec
2004, p. 339.

Espinal-Perez, L., et al. A double-blind randomized trial of 5% ascorbic acid vs.
4% hydroquinone in melasma. Int J Dermatol 43:604–7, 2004.

Facci, L., et al. Corticotropin-releasing factor (CRH) and related peptides confer neu-
roprotection via type 1 CRF receptors. Neuropharmacology 45:623–36, 2003.

Field, T., et al. Lavender fragrance cleansing gel effects on relaxation. Int
J Neurosci 115:207–22, 2005.

Fitton, A., and Goa, K. Azelaic acid. A review of its pharmacological properties
and therapeutic efficacy in acne and hyperpigmentary skin disorders. Drugs
41:780–98, 1991.

Fitzpatrick, R., and Rostan, E. Reversal of photodamage with topical growth factors: a pilot study. J Cosmet Laser Ther 5:25–34, 2003.

Frosch, P., and Kligman, A. The chamber-scarification test for irritancy. Contact
Dermatitis 2:314–24, 1976.

———. The soap chamber test. J Am Acad Dermatol 1:35–41, 1979.

Gallagher, R., et al. Tanning beds, sunlamps, and risk of cutaneous malignant
melanoma. Cancer Epidemiol Biomarkers Prev 14:562–66, 2005.

Garcia, A., and Fulton, J. The combination of glycolic acid and hydroquinone or
kojic acid for the treatment of melasma and related conditions. Dermatol
Surg 22:443–47, 1996.

Garg, A., et al. Psychological stress perturbs epidermal permeability barrier
homeostasis. Arch Dermatol 137:53–59, 2001.

Genuth, S., et al. Glycation and carboxymethyllysine levels in skin collagen predict the risk of future 10-year progression of diabetic retinopathy and
nephropathy in the diabetes control and complications trial and epidemiology of diabetes interventions and complications participants with type 1 diabetes. Diabetes 54:3103–11, 2005.

Gomolin, I., et al. Older is colder: temperature range and variation in older people. J Am Geriatr Soc 53:2170–72, 2005.

Goulden, V. Guidelines for the management of acne vulgaris in adolescents. Paediatr Drugs 5:301–13, 2003.

Graf, J. Herbal anti-inflammatory agents for skin disease. Skin Therapy Lett 5:3–5, 2000.

Green, A., et al. Daily sunscreen application and betacarotene supplementation in prevention of basal-cell and squamous-cell carcinomas of the skin: a randomized controlled trial. Lancet 354:723–29, 1999.

Green, B., et al. Maltobionic acid, a plant-derived bionic acid for topical anti-aging. American Academy of Dermatology meeting, San Francisco, March 4–6, 2006.

Grimes, P., et al. The use of polyhydroxy acids (PHAs) in photoaged skin. Cutis 73:3–13, 2004.

———. Evaluating the risks and benefits of treatment modalities for hyperpigmentation. Supplement to Skin and Aging, Sep. 2005, pp. 1–22.

———. Evaluation of inherent differences in ethnic skin types and response to topical polyhydroxy acid (PHA) use. Publication from the NeoStrata Company, 2006.

Grossman, R. The role of dimethyl aminoethanol in cosmetic dermatology. Am J Clin Dermatol 6:39–47, 2005.

Guttman, C. Topical imiquimod improves cosmetic appearance of photoaged skin. Dermatology Times, Aug. 2006, pp. 30–31.

Haes, P., et al. 1,25-Dihydroxyvitamin D_3 and analogues protect primary human keratinocytes against UVB-induced DNA damage. J Photochem Photobiol B: Biol 78:141–48, 2005.

Hakozaki, T., et al. Niacinamide: reversibility of reduction of facial hyperpigmentation spots. J Am Acad Dermatol 52(3):169

Hanson, K., and Clegg, R. Observation and quantification, of ultraviolet-induced reactive oxygen species in *ex vivo* human skin. J Photochem Photobiol 76:57–63, 2002.

Harvell, J., and Maibach, H. Percutaneous absorption and inflammation in aged skin: a review. J Am Acad Dermatol 31(6): 1015–21, 1994.

Hedelund, L., et al. Skin rejuvenation using intense pulsed light: a randomized controlled split-face trial with blinded response evaluation. Arch Dermatol 142:985–90, 2006.

Henderson, C., et al. Sebum excretion rates in mothers and neonates. Br J Dermatol 142:110–11, 2000.

Hermanns, J. Assessment of topical hypopigmenting agents on solar lentigines of Asian women. Dermatology 204:281–86, 2002.

Hillhouse, E. W., et al. Corticotropin-releasing hormone receptors. Biochem Soc Trans 30:428–32, 2002.

Humbert, P., et al. Ascorbic acid dermal concentration according to age. J Am Acad Dermatol 52(3): 26, 2005.

Isfort, R. J., et al. Discovery of corticotropin releasing factor 2 receptor selective sauvagine analogues for treatment of skeletal muscle atrophy. J Med Chem 48:262–65, 2005.

Jablonski, N. Skin: a natural history. Berkeley: University of California Press, 2006.

Jeanmaire, C., et al. Glycation during human dermal intrinsic and actinic ageing: an *in vivo* and *in vitro* model study. Br J Dermatol 145:10–18, 2001.

Jesitus, J. Ethnic skin: handle with care. Cosmetic Surgery Times, June 2004, pp. 1–2.

Juenst, E., et al. Antiaging research and the need for public dialogue. Science 299:1323, 2003.

Kakita, L., and Lowe, N. Azelaic acid and glycolic acid combination therapy for facial hyperpigmentation in darker-skinned patients: a clinical comparison with hydroquinone. Clin Ther 20:960–70, 1998.

Kameyama, K., et al. Inhibitory effect of magnesium L-ascorbyl-2-phosphate (VC-PMG) on melanogenesis *in vitro* and *in vivo*. J Am Acad Dermatol 34:29–33, 1996.

Karimipour, D., et al. Microdermabrasion: a molecular analysis following a single treatment. J Am Acad Dermatol 52:215–23, 2005.

Kaur, M., et al. Induction of withdrawal-like symptoms by opioid blockade in frequent tanners. J Am Acad Dermatol 54(4): 709–11, 2006

Kellett, N., et al. Conjoint analysis: a novel rigorous tool for determining patient preferences for topical antibiotic treatment for acne. Br J Dermatol 154:524–32, 2006.

Kligman, A. Cosmeceuticals. Dermatol Clin 18:609–15, 2000.

Kompaore, F., and Tsuruta H. *In vivo* differences between Asian, black and white in the stratum corneum barrier function. Int Arch Occup Environ Health 65:S223–25, 1993.

Kraus, E., et al. Effects of a melanogenic bicyclic monoterpene diol on cell cycle, p53, TNFa, and PGE$_2$ are distinct from those of UVB. Photodermatol Photoimmunol Photomed 19:295–302, 2003.

Kripke, M., et al. Pyrimidine dimers in DNA initiate systemic immunosuppression in UV-irradiated mice. Proc Natl Acad Sci USA 89:7516–20, 1992.

Kristjansoon, S., et al. The importance of assessing the readiness of changing sun-protection behaviour: a population-based study. Eur J Cancer 40: 2773–80, 2004.

Krutmann, J., and Yarosh, D. Modern photoprotection of human skin. In Gilchrist, B., and Krutman, J. Skin Aging. New York: Springer, 2006.

Larson, E., et al. Short- and long-term effects of handwashing with antimicrobial or plain soap in the community. J Community Health 28:139–50, 2003.

Lee, I., et al. Vitamin E in the primary prevention of cardiovascular disease and cancer: the Women's Health Study, a randomized controlled trial. JAMA 294:56–65, 2005.

Lewis, K., et al. Identification of urocortin III, an additional member of the corticotropin-releasing factor (CRF) family with high affinity for the CRF2 receptor. Proc Natl Acad Sci USA 98:7570–75, 2001.

Lombard, D., et al. DNA repair, genome stability, and aging. Cell 120:497–512, 2005.

Lou, W., et al. Effects of topical vitamin K and retinol on laser-induced purpura on nonlesional skin. Dermatol Surg 25:942–44, 1999.

Lowe, N., et al. Azelaic acid 20% cream in the treatment of facial hyperpigmentation in darker-skinned patients. Clin Ther 20:945–59, 1998.

Madison, K. Barrier function of the skin. J Invest Dermatol 121:23–41, 2003.

Maeda, K., and Fukuda, M. Arbutin: mechanism of its depigmenting action in human melanocytes culture. J Pharmacol Exp Ther 276:765–69, 1996.

Manton, K., et al. Long-term trends in life expectancy and active life expectancy in the United States. Popul Dev Rev 32:81–106, 2006.

Manziello, E. Kissed by the sun. Today's Health and Wellness, June/July 2006, pp. 26–28.

Marsee, K., et al. Estimated daily phthalate exposures in a population of mothers of male infants exhibiting reduced anogenital distance. Environ Health Perspect 114:805–9, 2006.

Mazur, A. W., et al. Determinants of corticotropin-releasing factor. Receptor selectivity of corticotropin-releasing factor related peptides. J Med Chem 47:3450–54, 2004.

McConnel, C., and Turner, L. Medicine, ageing and human longevity. EMBO Rep 6:S59–62, 2005.

Meerwaldt, R., et al. Skin autofluorescence, a measure of cumulative metabolic stress and advanced glycation end products, predicts mortality in hemodialysis patients. J Am Soc Nephrol 16:3687–93, 2005.

Melling, M., et al. Differential scanning calorimetry, biochemical, and biomechanical analysis of human skin from individuals with diabetes mellitus. Anat Rec 259:327–33, 2000.

Messina, M., et al. Addressing the soy and breast cancer relationship. J Natl Cancer Inst 98:1275–84, 2006.

Mignogna, G., et al. Tachykinins and other biologically active peptides from the skin of the Costa Rican phyllomedusid frog Agalychnis callidryas. Peptides 18:367–72, 1997.

Mills, O., et al. Comparing 2.5%, 5%, and 10% benzoyl peroxide on inflammatory acne vulgaris. Int J Dermatol 25:664–67, 1986.

Mozaffarian, D. Does alpha-linolenic acid intake reduce the risk of coronary heart disease? Altern Ther Health Med 11:24–30, 2005.

Nakagawa, M., et al. Contact allergy to kojic acid in skin care products. Contact Dermatitis 32:9–13, 1995.

Naylor, M., et al. High sun protection factor sunscreens in the suppression of actinic neoplasia. Arch Dermatol 131:170–75, 1995.

Nishimura, E., et al. Mechanisms of hair graying: incomplete melanocyte stem cell maintenance in the niche. Science 307:720–24, 2005.

Nusgens, B. V., et al. Topically applied vitamin C enhances the mRNA level of collagens I and III, their processing enzymes and tissue inhibitor matrix metalloproteinase 1 in the human dermis. J Invest Dermatol 116:853–59, 2001.

Obayashi, K., et al. L-ergothioneine scavenges superoxide and singlet oxygen and suppresses TNFa and MMP-1 expression in UV-irradiated human dermal fibroblasts. J Cosmet Sci 56:17–27, 2005.

O'Brien, L., and Pandit, A. Silicon gel sheeting for preventing and treating hypertrophic and keloid scars. Cochrane Database Syst Rev (1):CD003826, Jan. 25, 2006.

Off, M., et al. Ultraviolet photodegradation of folic acid. J Photochem Photobiol 80:47–55, 2005.

Ou-Yang, H., et al. A chemiluminescence study of UVA-induced oxidative stress in human skin *in vivo*. J Invest Dermatol 122:1020–29, 2004.

Ozolins M., et al. Randomised controlled multiple treatment comparison to provide a cost-effectiveness rationale for the selection of antimicrobial therapy in acne. Health Technol Assess 9:iii–212, 2005.

Pillai, S. et al. Structural homology of corticotropin-releasing factor, sauvagine, and urotensin I: circular dichroism and prediction studies. Proc Natl Acad Sci USA 80:6770–74, 1983.

––––––. Ultraviolet radiation and skin aging: roles of reactive oxygen species, inflammation and protease activation, and strategies for prevention of inflammation-induced matrix degradation—a review. Int J Cosmet Sci 27:17–34, 2005.

Prentice, R., et al. Low-fat dietary pattern and risk of invasive breast cancer: the Women's Health Initiative Randomized Controlled Dietary Modification Trial. JAMA 295:629–42, 2006.

Pugh, N., et al. Characterization of Aloeride, a new high-molecular-weight polysaccharide from aloe with potent immunostimulatory activity. J Agric Food Chem 49:1030–34, 2001.

Quatresooz, P. Cellulite histopathology and related mechanobiology. Int J Cosmet Sci 28:207–10, 2006.

Rabe J., et al. Photoaging: mechanisms and repair. J Am Acad Dermatol 55:1–19, 2006.

Rawlings, A. Trends in stratum corneum research and the management of dry skin conditions. Int J Cosmet Sci 25:63–95, 2003.

———. Ethnic skin types: are there differences in skin structure and function? Int J Cosmet Sci 28:79–94, 2006.

Rawlings, A., and Matts, P. Stratum corneum moisturization at the molecular level. J Invest Dermatol 124:1099–110, 2005.

Redoules, D., et al. Slow internal release of bioactive compounds under the effect of skin enzymes. J Invest Dermatol 125:270–77, 2005.

Rees, J. The melanocortin 1 receptor (MC1R): more than just red har. Pigment Cell Res 13:135–40, 2000.

———. Genetics of hair and skin colour. Annu Rev Genet 37:67–90, 2003.

———. The genetics of sun sensitivity in humans. Am J Hum Genet 75:739–51, 2004.

Reiser, K. M. Nonenzymatic glycation of collagen in aging and diabetes. Proc Soc Exp Biol Med 196:17–29, 1991.

Retiveau, A., et al. Common and specific effects of fine fragrances on the mood of women. J Sens Stud 19:373, 2004.

Rivas M. P., and Nouri, K. Temporary tissue fillers: a review. J Cosmet Dermatol 18:465–69, 2005.

Roney, J., et al. Reading men's faces: women's mate attractiveness judgments track men's testosterone and interest in infants. Proc R Soc Lond B Biol Sci 273:2169–75, 2006.

Samaha, F. Effect of very high-fat diets on body weight, lipoproteins, and glycemic status in the obsese. Curr Atheroscler Rep 7:412–20, 2005.

Samuel, M., et al. Interventions for photodamaged skin. Cochrane Database Syst Rev 1:CD001782, Jan. 25, 2005.

Sanghavi, D. Factors linked to a risk of early puberty. International Herald Tribune, Oct. 19, 2006, p. 9.

Sarkar, R., et al. A comparative study of 20% azelaic acid cream monotherapy versus a sequential therapy in the treatment of melasma in dark-skinned patients. Dermatology 205:249–54, 2002.

Saul, A., et al. Chronic stress and susceptibility to skin cancer. J Natl Cancer Inst 97:1760–67, 2005.

Scancarella, N., et al. Composition and method for under-eye skin lightening. US Patent 5,643,587, issued July 1, 1997.

Schmid, D., and Zülli, F. Mutations in mitochondrial DNA as principal aging factor. Cosmetics and Toiletries 122:71–76, 2007.

Slominski, A. On the role of melatonin in skin physiology and pathology. Endocrine 27:137–48, 2005.

Slominski, A., et al. Corticotropin-releasing hormone and related peptides can act as bioregulatory factors in human keratinocytes. In Vitr Cell Dev Biol Anim 36:211–16, 2000.

Smagin, G., et al. The role of CRh in behavioral responses to stress. Peptides 22:713–24, 2001.

Smeets, M., and Dalton, P. The nose of the beholder. The Aroma-Chology Review 8:1–12, 1999.

Soma, Y., et al. Moisturizing effects of topical nicotinamide on atopic dry skin. Int J Dermatol 44:197–202, 2005.

Sreekumaran, K., et al. DHEA in elderly women and DHEA or testosterone in elderly men. New Engl J Med 355:1647–59, 2006.

Stefánsson, H. The science of ageing and anti-ageing. EMBO Rep 6:S1–3, 2005.

Swan, S., et al. Decrease in anogenital distance among male infants with prenatal phthalate exposure. Environ Health Perspect 113:1056–61, 2005.

Thieden, E., et al. Proportion of lifetime UV dose received by children, teenagers and adults based on time-stamped personal dosimetry. J Invest Dermatol 123:1147–50, 2004.

Thiele, J. Oxidative targets in the stratum corneum. Skin Pharmacol Appl Skin Physiol 14(suppl):87–91, 2001.

Thiele, J., et al. The antioxidant network of the stratum corneum. Curr Probl Dermatol 29:26–42, 2001.

Thomas-Ahner, J., et al. Gender differences in UVB-induced skin carcinogenesis, inflammation, and DNA damage. Cancer Res 67:3468–74, 2007.

Thompson, S., et al. Reduction of solar keratoses by regular sunscreen use. New Engl J Med 329:1147–51, 1993.

Trommer, H., et al. Role of ascorbic acid in stratum corneum lipid models exposed to UV irradiation. Pharmacol Res 19:982–91, 2002.

Tuchinda, C., et al. Photoprotection by window glass, automobile glass, and sunglasses. J Am Acad Dermatol 54:845–54, 2006.

Uhodo, I., et al. Split face study on the cutaneous tensile effect of 2-dimethylaminoethanol (deanol) gel. Skin Res Technol 8:164–67, 2002.

Vasan, S. et al. Therapeutic potential of breakers of advanced glycation end product–protein crosslinks. Arch Biochem Biophys 419:89–96, 2003.

Verallo-Rowell, V., et al. Double-blind comparison of azelaic acid and hydroquinone in the treatment of melasma. Acta Derm Venereol Suppl (Stockh) 143:58–61, 1989.

Verzijl, N., et al. Effect of collagen turnover on the accumulation of advanced glycation end products. J Biol Chem 275:39027–31, 2000.

Wei, Q., et al. Association between low dietary folate intake and suboptimal cellular DNA repair capacity. Cancer Epidemiology Biomarkers, Prev 12:963–69, 2003.

Weil, A. Healthy aging. New York: Alfred A. Knopf, 2005.

Wolf, P., et al. Effects of sunscreens and a DNA excision repair enzyme on ultraviolet radiation–induced inflammation, immune suppression, and cyclobutane pyrimidine dimer formation. J Invest Dermatol 101:523–27, 1993.

Yarosh, D. The molecular biology of aging. Chem Innov 30:21–24, 2000.

———. DNA repair, immunosuppression, and skin cancer. Cutis 74(5S):10–13, 2004.

Yarosh, D., et al. Cyclobutane pyrimidine dimer removal enhanced by DNA repair liposomes reduces the incidence of UV skin cancer in mice. Cancer Res 52:4227–37, 1992.

———. Enzyme therapy of xeroderma pigmentosum: safety and efficacy testing of T4N5 liposome lotion containing a prokaryotic DNA repair enzyme. Photodermatol Photoimmunol Photomed 12:122–39, 1996.

———. Effect of topically applied T4 endonuclease V in liposomes on skin cancer in xeroderma pigmentosum: a randomized study. Lancet 357:926–29, 2001.

———. After sun reversal of DNA damage: enhancing skin repair. Mutat Res 571:57–64, 2005.

———. Anti-inflammatory activity in skin by biomimetic of *Evodia rutaecarpa* extract from traditional Chinese medicine. J Dermatol Sci 42:13–21, 2006.

Yokota, T., et al. The inhibitory effect of glabridin from licorice extracts on melanogenesis and inflammation. Pigment Cell Res 11:355–61, 1998.

Zangwill, M. Nonmelanoma skin cancer: saving your skin. Cure, Summer 2006, p. 43.

Zeller, S., et al. Do adolescent indoor tanners exhibit dependency? J Am Acad Dermatol 54:589–96, 2006.

Zhao, X., et al. DNA protection from supplemental carotenoid mixture intake (Excerpt). Am J Clin Nutr 83:51, 2006.

Zouboulis, C. Acne and sebaceous gland function. Clin Dermatol 22:360–66, 2004.

Zurada, J., et al. Topical treatments for hypertrophic scars. J Am Acad Dermatol 55:1024–31, 2006.

INDEX

Accutane, 252
Acetyl hexapeptide-3, 208–9
Acne
    prescription drugs for, 251–52
    product ingredients to avoid,
        252–53
    recommended products for, 269–70
    skin-care regimens for, 249–53
Actinic keratosis, 151
Adapalene, 200
Advertorials, 57
Aftershaves, 254–55
AGE (advanced glycation end-products),
    209–10
Age spots, 165–66
AGI Dermatics, 1
Aging's impact on skin, 16–21, 25–28
AHAs (alpha-hydroxy acids), 63, 203–5,
    221
Airless pump bottles, 46
Alberto VO5 hair-care products, 2
Albinos, 155
Aloe, 103, 147
Alpha-lipoic acid, 185–86
Animal-derived ingredients, 78
Antibiotics, topical, 252
Anti-inflammatories, 102–4
Antimicrobial cleansers, 89–91
Antioxidants, 62
    DNA repair and, 192

exfoliation and, 188–89, 204–5
in foods, 178–79
free radical theory of aging and,
    174–78
how and when to use, 190–92
isoflavones, 194–95
in New Skin-Care Revolution
    products, 187–90, 192–95
overhyped antioxidant ingredients,
    182, 184–87
recommended products, 189, 190,
    191–92, 193–94, 195, 264–66
in skin, 178, 182
in standard skin-care products,
    181–84
sun protection and, 182, 186–87
sunscreens and, 191–92
in supplements, 23, 179–81
"team" approach to using, 188–90
See also Ergothioneine
Arabidopsis extract, 69
Arbutin, 167, 172
Argireline, 208–9
Aromatherapy
    holistic medicine and, 236
    moisturizers and, 108–9
    recommended products, 269
Ascorbic acid, 170
Astringents, 92
Avage, 200

Avobenzone, 128, 129
Azelaic acid, 168–69

Bacterial contamination of skin-care
    products, 45–46, 75–77
Baldness treatments, 255, 256
Basal cell carcinoma (BCC), 151
Beer, Kenneth R., 208, 210
Before-and-after photos, 50–52
Benzoyl peroxide, 251
Beta-carotene, 179, 180, 181
BHAs (beta-hydroxy acids), 64, 204
Bisabolol, 103
Black, Homer, 179
Blake, Milton, 125
Blanching reaction, 175
Blood circulation, 105–7
Boscia Daily Hand Revival Therapy, 72
Boswelox, 211
Botanical extracts
    anti-inflammatories, 103–4
    brighteners/lighteners, 170–71
    commonly used extracts, 70–71
    essences, 72–73
    future products, 231–32
    potency of, 73–75
    "preservative free" issue, 76–77
    sun protection and, 140
Botox injections, 218, 219–20
    peptide treatments, comparison with,
        208–9
Brash, Douglas, 186
Brighteners/lighteners, 39
    age spots and, 165–66
    alternate products, 168–70
    ingredients in, 64
    laser treatments, 229
    New Skin-Care Revolution products,
        171–73
    products to avoid, 170–71
    recommended products, 168, 169,
        172, 173, 267–68
    tried and true products, 166–68
Bronzing-booth tanning, 162–63

Bronzing makeup, 163–64
Brown spots, 120

Caffeine, 111
Calming agents, 62–63, 102–4
Camphanediol, 69
Cancer. See Skin cancer
Captique, 225
Carnitine, 106, 112
Cat's claw, 145
Cellulite, 110–12
Ceramides, 15, 19, 113
Chamomile, 103
Chanel, Coco, 124
Chelation therapy, 114
Chemical peels, 217, 221
Chesebrough, Robert, 94–95
Childbearing years, 17–18
Children's skin-care needs, 249
Chinese medicine for skin, 72
Chloasma (mask of pregnancy), 166
Cleansers, 83
    antimicrobial cleansers, 89–91
    detergents, 84–85
    finding the best cleanser for you, 86–87
    ingredients in, 63, 68
    ingredients to avoid, 93
    irritants in, 68
    proper use of, 85–86
    purpose of a cleansing regimen,
        83–84
    recommended cleansers with added
        ingredients, 259
    recommended daytime cleansers, 87,
        258
    recommended nighttime cleansers,
        88–89, 258
    soaps, 84–85, 87
"Clinically proven" claims, 39–40
Clinical testing of skin-care products,
    52–55
Clothing for sun protection, 130–31,
    135–36
Collagen, 14, 19, 197–98

Collagenase, 122–23
Collagen builders, 111–12
Collagen fillers, 224–25, 226
Color of skin
    color-related problems, 157–59
    melanin and, 155–56, 159, 161
    variations among ethnic groups, 156–57
    See also Brighteners/lighteners; Tanning
Contraceptive use and skin
    discoloration, 166
Copper peptides, 113–14, 208
Coppertone sunscreen, 125–26
CoQ10, 47–48
Cosmeceuticals, 36–37, 232
Cosmetics, 34–36
CosmoDerm and CosmoPlast, 225
CO$_2$ (carbon dioxide) lasers, 227–28
Creams, 96
Creatine, 145
Curél Age Defying Therapeutic
    Moisturizing Lotion, 47
Cytokines, 122, 123
Cytokinins, 114

Dark under-eye circles, 107–10
Deep-tissue massage, 111
Denese, Adrienne, 112
Deodorant soaps, 87
Dermatologists, 232–33
"Dermatologist tested and
    recommended" claims, 40
Dermis, 14–15
Detergents, 84–85
"Detoxifying" claims, 40
DHA (dihydroacetone), 161
Diabetes, 24
Diet, 22–25, 237–38
Differin, 200
Dimericine, 141–42
Dinoire, Isabelle, 220
Diol cream, 109–10
DMAE (dimethylaminoethanol), 211–12
DNA damage due to sun exposure,
    120–23

DNA fragments to trigger tanning
    response, 164
DNA program of skin, 15–16, 18–19
DNA repair, 3–4, 7, 16, 25–28
    antioxidants and, 192
    gene therapy for skin, 233–35
    ingredients for, 67–68
    recommended products, 259–62
    sun protection and, 118, 139–47
Doctors' patient studies, 53
Doctor treatments
    Botox injections, 218, 219–20
    face-lifts, 217–18
    injectable fillers, 223–26
    IPL (intense pulsed light), 222–23
    lasers and other light treatments, 111,
        158, 226–28, 229
    peels, 217, 221–22
    radiofrequency treatments, 111,
        228–30
    shortcomings of, 218
Double-blind, placebo-controlled
    studies, 53
"Dusting" of skin-care products, 47–48,
    185

ECGC, 182–83
Eczema, 119
Efudex, 153
Elastase, 122–23
Elastin, 14, 197–98, 202
Epidermis, 14, 15
Ergothioneine, 69
    as antioxidant, 190, 193–94
    as brightener, 172
    in moisturizers, 106–7
Essential oils, 108–9
Eumelanin, 155, 159
Evodia extract, 69
Evolence, 226
Exfoliation
    AHA and PHA exfoliants, 63–64,
        203–5
    antioxidants and, 188–89, 204–5

lasers and other light treatments, 226–28, 229
peels, 217, 221–22
recommended products, 266
Eyeseryl, 209–10

Face-lifts, 217–18
Facial expressions, 220
Factor, Max, 2
Fibroblasts, 14
Fillers, 223–26
"Firming/lifting" claims, 40
Folic acid, 145
Food, Drug, and Cosmetic Act of 1938, 35
Fragrances
holistic medicine and, 235–36
irritation from, 69
Fraxel SR laser, 228
Free radical theory of aging, 174–78
Free samples, 38
Freeze 24-7 products, 212–13
Future of skin care, 231–39

GABA (gamma-aminobutyric acid), 212–13
Galumbeck, Matthew, 213
Gels, 96
Gene therapy for skin, 233–35
Genistein, 194
Glycation, 209–10
Glycolic acid, 203–4
Glycyrrhizinate, 171
Green, Benjamin, 125
Green tea, 147, 182–83
Gross, Dennis F., 114

Hair removal, 223
Harman, Denham, 176–77
Hats for sun protection, 135–36
Healthy Aging (Weil), 42
Herbal medicine, 72

Hertz, Kenneth, 186
Holistic medicine, 78, 80, 235–36
Humectants, 95, 96
Hyaluronic acid, 225, 226
Hydrogen peroxide, 175
Hydroquinone, 167–68
Hylaform, 225
Hyperpigmentation, 120, 229
"Hypoallergenic" claims, 40

Idebenone, 186–87
Imaging systems, 236–37
Imiquimod, 153, 158
Immune system
baldness and, 255
inflammation and, 102
products for immune enhancement, 147–48
sun exposure, damage from, 123–24
Inflammation, 102–4
Infomercials, 57
Ingredients in skin-care products, 58–59
active ingredients, 59–60
animal-derived ingredients, 78
botanical extracts, 70–75
"holistic" concerns, 78, 80
ingredients to look for, 62–68
irritants, 68–69
label information about, 59–62
natural and organic ingredients, 77–78, 80
patented ingredients, 76
preservatives, 75–77
IPF (immune protection factor), 239
IPL (intense pulsed light) treatments, 222–23
Irritants, 68–69, 115–16
Isoflavones, 194–95
Isotretinoin, 252

Jars as containers, 45–46
Jessner's peel, 221
Juvéderm, 226

Kelner, Albert, 142
Keloids, 158
Keratinocytes, 15
Kinetin, 114
Kligman, Albert, 199
Kojic acid, 169

Lactic acid, 203–4
Laser treatments, 111, 158, 226–28, 229
Leffell, David, 186
Lerner, Aaron, 171
Licorice, 103
Licorice root extract, 171
Lighteners. See Brighteners/lighteners
Lip balms, 96
Lipolysis, 111
Liposomes, 140–41
Lip plumpers, 215
Liquid nitrogen peels, 221–22
Liver spots, 165–66
Lotions, 96

Magnetic microparticles in cosmetics, 106
MAP (magnesium ascorbyl phosphate), 170, 202
Marketing of skin-care products, 31–32, 38–41, 49–52, 57
Mask of pregnancy (chloasma), 166
"Mastige" market, 48
Matrixyl, 210
Media coverage of skin-care products, 55–56
Medicis Pharmaceutical Corporation, 76
Melanin, 155–56, 159, 161
Melanoma, 152
Melanotan tanning agent, 164
Melasma, 158
Melatonin, 171
Menopause, 19
Men's skin care, 253–56
  recommended products, 256, 270

Menstruation, 18
Metered dispensers, 46
Methylparaben, 79
Methylxanthines, 111
Mexoryl SX, 130
Micrococcus lysate, 69
Microdermabrasion, 222
Microscars, 122, 198
Middle-age years, 18–19
Minoxidil, 255
Mitochondrial DNA, 192
MMP enzymes, 144, 198, 213–14
Mohs surgery, 153
Moisturizers, 2
  anti-inflammatories, 102–4
  aromatherapy and, 108–9
  blood circulation and, 105–7
  B vitamins, 101–2
  cellulite reduction and, 110–12
  collagen builders, 111–12
  for dark under-eye circles, 107–10
  with ergothioneine, 106–7
  history of, 94–95
  how basic moisturizers work, 95–97
  ingredients for moisturizing, 64–65
  ingredients to avoid, 112–16
  irritants in, 69, 115–16
  for men, 254
  power moisturizers, 99–112
  recommended products, 97–99, 101–2, 104, 107, 109, 110, 112, 259–62
  steroids, 104–5
  with sunscreen, 97–98, 133–34
  toners, 92
  types of, 96–97
  ursolic acid, 100–101
Multitasking products, 237
Mystic Tan Tanning Myst, 163

"Natural" diet, 23–24
Natural ingredients, 77–78, 80
Neuropeptides, 114–15
Neurotransmitters, 22

New Skin-Care Revolution, 1–4
Niacin, 145–46
Niacinamide, 101–2
Nitric oxide, 109–10
"Noncomedogenic" claims, 40
Norbordiol tanning agent, 165
Nutrition, 22–25
Nutritional cosmetics, 237–38

OGG1 enzyme, 192
"Oil free" claims, 40–41
Onchronosis, 167
Organic ingredients, 77–78, 80
Osteoporosis, 138
Over-the-counter (OTC) products,
    32–34

PABA chemical filter, 126
Panthenol, 101–2
Parabens, 79
Parsol 1789, 128, 129
Patented ingredients, 76
Peels, 217, 221–22
Peptides, 206–10
Perricone, Nicholas, 22, 76, 112, 114,
    185, 196, 212
Petroleum jelly, 94–95, 96
PHAs (polyhydroxy acids), 64, 204–5
Phenol peels, 221
Pheomelanin, 155, 159
Photoaging, 17, 117, 197–98
Photolyase, 142–43
Photoreactivation, 142
Phthalates, 79
Phytoestrogens, 194–95
Pinanediol, 69
Placebo effect, 53
Plant estrogens, 194–95
Plastic surgeons, 232–33
Poikiloderma, 166
Poly-L-lactic acid, 225–26
Polymorphisms, 234
Polypeptide 153, 210

Pregnancy, 18, 166
Preservatives, 75–77
Preventive approach to skin care, 233
Pricing of skin-care products, 46–48
Probiotic Anti-Stress Lotion, 91
Pro-oxidants, 180
Propecia, 255
Psoriasis, 22, 119
PSR 3 high-energy plasma device,
    229–30
Pumps for dispensing skin-care
    products, 46

Radiesse, 226
Radiofrequency treatments, 111, 228–30
Regimens. See Skin-care regimens
Remergent skin-care products, 1
Renova, 200
Restylane, 225
Retin-A, 199–200, 252
Retinoic acid
    in anti-acne drugs, 252
    as antioxidant, 184
    as brightener, 169–70
    as wrinkle treatment, 199–200
Retinol
    as antioxidant, 184
    as brightener, 169–70
    as wrinkle treatment, 200–201
Rickets, 138
Rigel, Darrell S., 132
Rosemary extract, 74, 78, 100

Salicylic acid, 250–51
Schueller, Eugène, 125
Scientific claims about skin-care
    products, 52–55
Sculptra, 225–26
Seaweed, 47, 146
Selenium, 146–47, 181
Senior years, 20–21
Sepiwhite, 172–73
Serums, 96–97

Side-by-side studies, 53–54
Skin
  aging's impact on, 16–21, 25–28
  antioxidant system of, 178, 182
  blood supply for, 105–6
  diet and, 22–25, 237–38
  evolutionary perspective on, 13–14,
    18–19
  physiology of, 14–16
  sex and, 13–14
  stress and, 21–22
  sunburn cells in, 186–87
  sun exposure, damage from, 17, 117,
    120–24, 197–98
Skin cancer
  beta-carotene and, 179
  causes of, 121, 150–51
  immune system and, 123–24
  self-examination for, 152–53
  solar lentigines and, 165–66
  statistics on, 150
  stress and, 22
  tanning and, 159–61
  treatment of, 141–42, 153
  types of, 151–52
  XP disease and, 141–42
Skin-care products
  amount of product inside a container,
    43
  bacterial contamination concerns,
    45–46, 75–77
  before-and-after photos about, 50–52
  brand loyalty and, 37–38
  confusion regarding, 4–7
  containers and how they work, 45–46
  cosmeceuticals, 36–37, 232
  cosmetics, 34–36
  false claims by manufacturers, 49–55
  free samples, 38
  future products, 231–39
  information inserts, 45
  instructions for use, 44–45
  laws concerning, 35–36
  luxury and drug store products, 8
  manufacturer's reputation, 41–42

  marketing of, 31–32, 38–41, 49–52,
    57
  media coverage of, 55–56
  over-the-counter products, 32–34
  package information about, 42–48
  pricing of, 46–48
  product recommendations in this
    book, 9
  scientific claims about, 52–55
  third-millennium products, 3–4
  verbal messages about, 50
  visual messages about, 49
  See also Ingredients in skin-care
    products; *specific products*
Skin-care regimens
  basic regimens, 243–48
  for children, 249
  evening regimen, 245–48
  fewer products used, benefits of, 34
  morning regimen, 244–45, 246–48
  new products, incorporation of, 37
  sample regimens, 246–48
  for teenagers with acne, 249–53
  wrinkle cream application, 214–16
Skin color. *See* Color of skin
SNAP-25 protein, 208–9
Soaps, 84–85, 87
Solar lentigines, 165–66
SPF (sun protection factor), 126–28,
  132
Spider veins, 223
Squamous cell carcinoma (SCC),
  151
Steroids, 104–5
Stratum corneum, 15, 19, 157, 204
Streilein, J. Wayne, 123
Stress, 21–22
Stress reducers, 269
Sunburn cells in skin, 186–87
Sun exposure
  damage to skin from, 17, 117,
    120–24, 197–98
  immune system and, 123–24
  inflammation and, 102
  statistics on, 150

UVA and UVB wavelengths of light,
118–20
wrinkles and, 197–98
See also Skin cancer
Sunlamps, 160–61
Sun protection, 117–18
antioxidants and, 182, 186–87
for children, 249
clothing and hats, 130–31, 135–36
DNA repair enzymes, 118, 139–44
DNA repair mystery ingredients,
144–47
future developments, 238–39
history of, 124–25
immune system and, 147–48
midday sun, avoidance of, 136
reasonable precautions, 148–49
recommended products, 144, 147,
148
See also Sunscreens
Sunscreens, 148–49
age-related concerns in use of, 137,
139
antioxidants and, 191–92
best sunscreens, 128–31
"broad spectrum" sunscreens, 126,
128
clothing, use on, 130–31
correct use of, 131–35
earliest sunscreens, 125–26
effective ingredients, 128–29
expiration dates, 134
future products, 239
ghosting effect, 126
health risks of using, 127–28, 138
ingredients in, 65–66
ingredients to avoid, 131
IPF (immune protection factor), 239
moisturizers with sunscreen, 97–98,
133–34
non-use of, 136–37
reapplication guidelines, 133
recommended products, 129, 130,
134–35, 263–64
regulations concerning, 132

safety-review Web site, 131
SPF (sun protection factor), 126–28,
132
spray sunscreens, 134–35
UVA and UVB filters, 65–66
vitamin D deficiency and, 138

Tamarind seeds, 148
Tanning
bronzing makeup, 163–64
DNA fragments to trigger tanning
response, 164
Melanotan tanning agent, 164
New Skin-Care Revolution products,
164–65
Norbordiol tanning agent, 165
recommended products, 162, 163–64,
268
self-tanning at home, 161–62
self-tanning in bronzing booth,
162–63
skin cancer and, 159–61
sunlamps and, 160–61
sunless tanning, 161–65
Tattoos, 156, 223
Tazarotene, 200
TCA (trichloroacetic acid), 221
Teenagers with acne, 249–53
TGF-beta, 214
ThermaCool radiofrequency device, 230
Tinosorb, 130–31
Titanium dioxide, 128–29
Titan laser, 228
Toners, 83, 91–93
astringents, 92
ingredients in, 66
ingredients to avoid, 93
moisturizing toners, 92
Tretinoin, 199–200
Triclosan, 90
Tropoelastin, 207
Tubes for dispensing skin-care products,
46
Tyrosinase, 155

University research on skin-care
    products, 54
Ursolic acid, 100–101
UVA and UVB wavelengths of light,
    65–66, 118–20
UV endonuclease, 143–44

Vitamin A
    as antioxidant, 180, 181, 183–84
    brighteners/lighteners and,
        169–70
    derivatives of, 60
    as wrinkle treatment, 199–201
Vitamin B
    moisturizing B vitamins, 101–2
    sun protection and, 145–46
Vitamin C
    as antioxidant, 180, 181, 183–84,
        190, 191
    brighteners/lighteners and, 170
    derivatives of, 60
    immune system and, 147
    in moisturizers, 106, 107
    as wrinkle treatment, 201–3
Vitamin D
    color of skin and, 156
    sunscreens and, 138
Vitamin E, 23
    as antioxidant, 180, 181, 183–84,
        190, 191

derivatives of, 60
immune system and, 147
Vitamin K, 107–8, 110
Vitamin therapy, 181
Vitiligo, 158
Voorhees, John, 224

Weil, Andrew, 42
Wexler, Patricia, 213
Wrinkles, causes of, 197–98
Wrinkle treatments, 196
    AHA and PHA exfoliants, 203–5
    how to use wrinkle creams,
        214–16
    ingredients in, 66–67
    peptides, 206–10
    recommended products, 201, 203,
        205
    unreliable products, 206–14
    vitamin A, 199–201
    vitamin C, 201–3
Wu Zhu Yu elixir, 103

XP (xeroderma pigmentosum),
    141–42

Zinc oxide, 128–29
Zyderm and Zyplast, 224

ABOUT THE AUTHOR

Daniel B. Yarosh, PhD, is widely recognized as a pioneer in the science of DNA repair and the development of cosmeceuticals. Following research appointments at the National Cancer Institute and Brookhaven National Laboratory, he founded the Long Island–based biopharmaceutical company AGI Dermatics. The ingredients Dr. Yarosh invented at AGI Dermatics are used by the most respected brands in the cosmetics industry, including Coty, Estée Lauder, and Shiseido. In 2004, Dr. Yarosh received the Finsen Award for his breakthrough research in photobiology. He is the author of more than one hundred scientific papers on the science of skin and DNA repair. His products and cosmetic innovations have been featured widely in the media, including *ABC World News Tonight*, *Wall Street Journal*, *Time*, *Newsweek*, *Vogue*, *Self*, *Allure*, *Prevention*, and *Good Housekeeping*, among others.